Wa

Causative Factors of
Ulcerative Colitis and Crohn's Disease

W.E.W. (Bill) Roediger is a clinical scientist who has researched ulcerative colitis and Crohn's disease for forty years using mainly patient-derived observations.

Causative Factors of Ulcerative Colitis and Crohn's Disease

An Exploratory Guide

BILL ROEDIGER

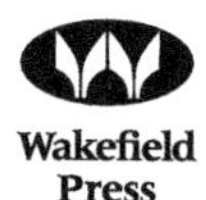

Wakefield Press
16 Rose Street
Mile End
South Australia 5031
www.wakefieldpress.com.au

First published 2016
Reprinted 2017

Copyright © W.E.W. Roediger, 2016

All rights reserved. This book is copyright. Apart from any fair dealing for the purposes of private study, research, criticism or review, as permitted under the Copyright Act, no part may be reproduced without written permission. Enquiries should be addressed to the publisher.

Cover: 'The Road Ahead', painting by Olga Konoschuk, Adelaide, South Australia, 2013. Reproduced with permission.

Designed and typeset by Wakefield Press

National Library of Australia Cataloguing-in-Publication entry

Creator:	Roediger, Bill, author.
Title:	Causative factors of ulcerative colitis and Crohn's disease: an exploratory guide / Bill Roediger.
ISBN:	978 1 74305 433 8 (paperback).
Subjects:	Ulcerative colitis. Crohn's disease.
Dewey Number:	616.344

CONTENTS

Acknowledgements viii

Preface xi

Introduction 1

PART 1 WAYS AND MEANS

1 Final conclusions about the causative factors of ulcerative colitis and Crohn's disease 5

2 The impetus and history of ulcerative colitis and Crohn's disease 8

3 The evolving philosophy of science and research of disease causation 11

PART 2 ULCERATIVE COLITIS

4 The biological compartments of the colon: concepts in man or animal? 17

5 Nutrient sustenance of colonic epithelial cells (colonocytes) 20

6 The biochemical lesions in colonocytes of ulcerative colitis 26

7 Agents causing the biochemical lesions in colonocytes of ulcerative colitis 33

8 Vascular and dietary sources of colonic nitrogen and sulphur 48

9 Slow toxicity and colonic extent of ulcerative colitis 51

10 Treatment of the precipitating factors of ulcerative colitis. The concept of bioremediation 54

11 Conclusions on the causation of ulcerative colitis – the strength of evidence 59

PART 3 CROHN'S DISEASE

12 A profusion of ideas for Crohn's disease 65

13 *Mycobacterium avium* subspecies *paratuberculosis* (MAP) 70

14 Enteric *Listeria monocytogenes* in Crohn's disease 74

15 Pathogenic *Escherichia coli* in Crohn's disease 77

16 *Mycoplasma* in the causation of Crohn's disease 80

17 Antibiotics in Crohn's disease: any clues? 93

PART 4 THE ROAD AHEAD

18 A communality of Colitis 99

19 Future research into the causation of ulcerative colitis and Crohn's disease 102

Appendix – Dietary treatment of ulcerative colitis 106

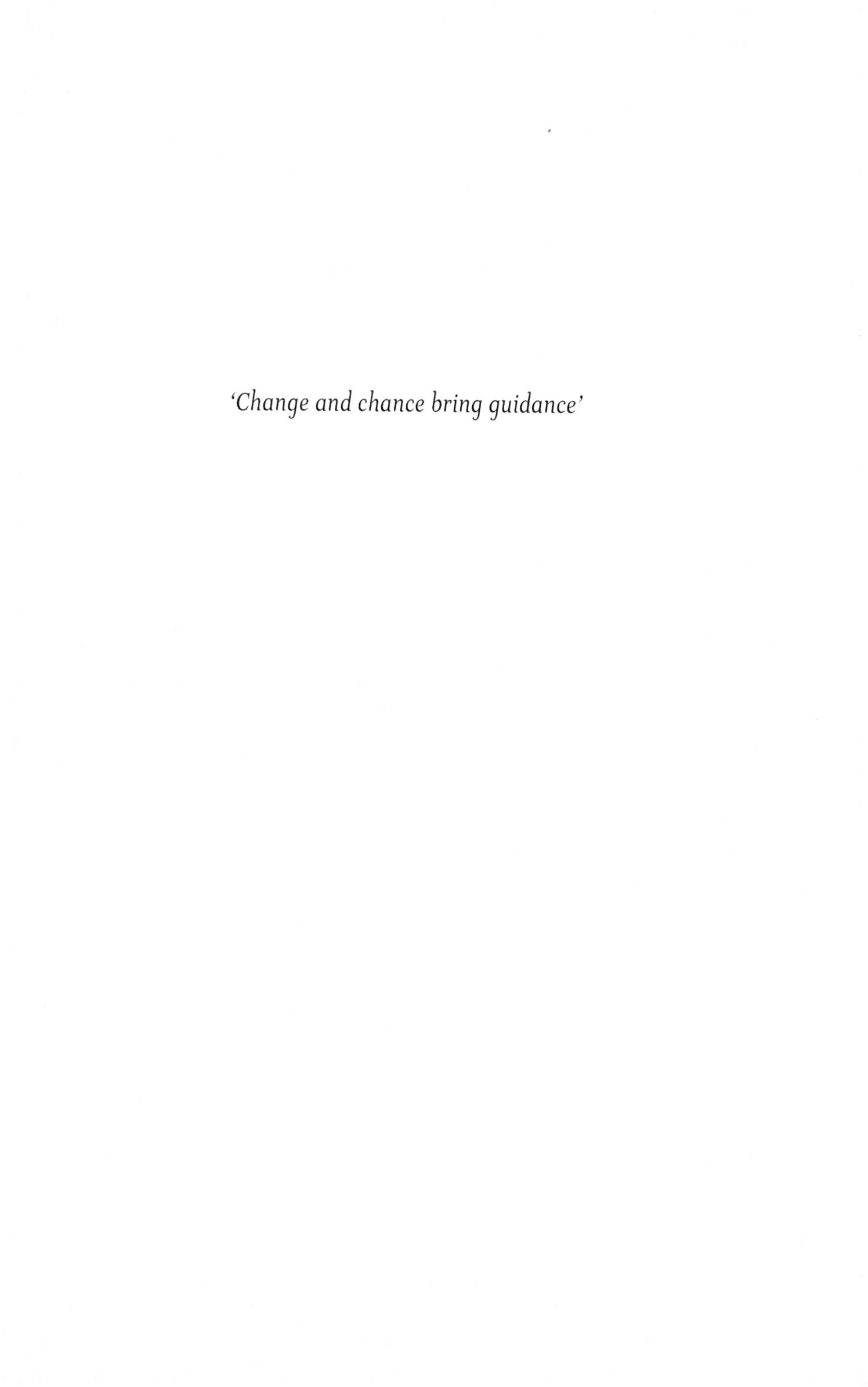

'Change and chance bring guidance'

Acknowledgements

Over many years, numerous clinicians and scientists, some of whom have sadly passed away, have helped me to research inflammatory bowel disease.

Firstly Issy Segal of Sydney was foremost in prodding me to write this book, probably through the impact of earlier studies on short chain fatty acids in the human colon. The new ideas, proposed then, were rebellious but correct. I am most grateful for his encouragements over the years.

Ann Andrew, Phillip Tobias, Sonny du Plessis and Buddy Lawson of the Medical School, University of the Witwatersrand, encouraged my youthful desires for conducting research. Huge thanks go to Tom Bothwell, whose Intern I was, and especially for his help to secure a Nuffield Dominions Trust Scholarship to Oxford to study under Sidney Truelove, Mani Lee, Hans Krebs and Peter Morris. All were most supportive and my heartfelt gratitude for their encouragements. Others in Oxford, particularly Dennis Parsons, Patricia Lund and Brian Ross were great encouragers, enabling me to do some daring experiments. I thank them all for support towards new ideas. David Weatherall permitted me to have a desk in the Nuffield Dept of Medicine thus enabling me to have one foot in a physician's world and the other in the surgical world under Peter Morris. Oliver Wrong from University College, London, and Paul Porteous from Aberdeen provided great advice.

The biochemical team of the Metabolic Research Laboratory in Oxford (Reg Hems, Pat Lund, Derek Williamson, David Wiggins and Geoff Gibbons) guided and helped in pursuing biochemical work according to the conventions of cell biochemistry.

A pillar of support came from Cambridge University, Dunn School of Nutrition, through help and numerous discussions with John Cummings, Glen Gibson and George McFarlane.

It was a chance encounter with Vernon Marshall in Brian Ross's laboratory in Oxford that began the road to Melbourne and Monash University. I am forever grateful to Paula Jablonski, Vernon Marshall and the Marshall dynasty in Melbourne who made research there possible.

Family connections, friends and surgery drew me to the University of Adelaide and the Queen Elizabeth Hospital. Ron Elmslie, Glyn Jamieson and Tony Slavotinek enabled ten productive years of laboratory and clinical research work. To them I am most grateful. Ron Elmslie had established a biochemical laboratory which needed new directions. This was achieved with the aid of Allen Kerr Grant, Ross Butler, Mike Lawson, Sue Millard, Barbara Radcliffe, Wendy Babidge, Prue Cowled and Elaine Deakin. The untramelled environment to find the causative agent of ulcerative colitis took all these years of work at the Queen Elizabeth Hospital. We were joined by James Moore who with his expertise hugely assisted in these endeavours. I would particularly like to thank George Gream, organic chemist at the University of Adelaide, who produced gram quantities of nitric oxide-donating agents through his synthetic wizardry.

Numerous granting bodies provided financial support, but especially the Australian National Health and Medical Research Council gave financial backing over 16 years. In this period Bill Doe and Graeme Young facilitated the work that led to the conclusions about the causative factors of ulcerative colitis outlined in this book.

Negative aspects of research endeavours are rarely acknowledged. Attempts to highlight an infective organism causing Crohn's disease were scientifically doubted for many years. Research grants on causative organisms were turned down, often for diaphanous reasons, even though reviewers applauded the ingenuity of the proposals made.

Of great value was a sympathetic ear given to our work by Ross Philpott, Ian Roberts-Thomson, Adrian Cummins, Dick Heddle and Derek Jewell. Some of these colleagues experienced the complete clinical restoration to health of cases of Crohn's disease treated by methods discussed in this book.

My very special thanks go to the reviewers of this book: Issy Segal, David Grove and Justin le Brooy. Their suggestions have been invaluable. My thanks go to Guy Maddern, who allowed me a length of stay in the Department of Surgery at The Queen Elizabeth Hospital.

The word processing skills of Ernesta Smythe, Debbie Seskis and further assistance by Sandra Ireland aided compilation. I am very grateful to them for their help and skills.

My gratitude to Michael Bollen and Michael Deves at Wakefield Press for bringing this book to life. Basil Popowycz used his computer wizardry to produce the cover design and the figures in the text. I owe him a great debt of thanks.

Finally, my family provided the life support for me that was in turn essential to help suffering patients. My children provided diversion when rejections of work proposals came through. They are a marvellous team.

Above all I hope that this research work has improved patients' health. This book is dedicated to them.

Preface

From clinical and experimental observations this book seeks a pathway to understanding the causation of ulcerative colitis and Crohn's disease. The narrative is not a check list of all the clinical, immunological, biochemical, genetic or microbiological abnormalities so far observed in either Crohn's disease or ulcerative colitis. Such information is readily obtainable from electronic search engines as well as published textbooks or reference books on inflammatory bowel disease. Selected themes of the book attempt to tease out a central path that leads to the causation of the disease processes of ulcerative colitis and Crohn's disease. Answers to certain questions, through experimentation, are provided and thereby proffered as a model of causation of inflammatory bowel disease. Inevitably good answers almost always raise further questions.

Throughout the chapters results derived from humans in health and disease are used, that is patient-based evidence, because animal experimentation infrequently determines human disease processes. Nevertheless animal experimentation may amplify observations taken from human disease in order to confirm that such biological processes could occur in mammalian tissues.

Chapters of the book have been kept short in line with the byte-sized information of modern electronic communications. Brevity sometimes necessitates selectivity particularly where incremental results may relate to the causation of inflammatory bowel disease. A drawn out analysis of multiple interpretations of reported observations was not undertaken.

New concepts, not previously publicised, are often difficult to incorporate into an established body of knowledge. The human mind in general prefers the security of tradition to the uncertainty of what is new. When William Harvey wrote *De Motu Cordis* (On the Motion of the Heart) in 1628 he was faced with a medical world steeped in the Galenic teaching of the passivity of the heart. Harvey's new idea could not safely be published in London, where he worked, but instead was printed in Frankfurt, Germany, in order to maintain medical peace in London. Consequent developments in physiology of the heart showed that the 'new' knowledge was not noise but the substrate of future progress.

The modern equivalent to Harvey's experience as applied to inflammatory bowel disease, is that ulcerative colitis and Crohn's disease have an immunocentric focus, putting other pathological possibilities aside. Immunological changes are prominent in inflammatory bowel disease but immune cell behaviour as the originator of the disease processes of inflammatory bowel disease is lacking. What happens before immune cells are activated in inflammatory bowel disease? The book attempts to answer this question and define those factors with which immune processes become closely involved. Attempts were made to think broadly and not just in one compartment of the gastro-intestinal tract.

This book may be considered a scientific biography of disease processes in ulcerative colitis and Crohn's disease. The proposed concepts have not received prime consideration in standard texts of inflammatory bowel disease. Prematurity of scientific reports and uniqueness of scientific discovery often presage processes that are later considered appropriate but only after a long period of neglect of pertinent observations. The current narrative recognises the limits of scientific knowledge: it is not a body of permanent truth but an amalgam of successive scientific approximations which provides understanding in a sea of mystery of two diseases. Hopefully this book will not provoke a backlash against the science of inflammatory bowel disease particularly as not every scientific discovery in the field of inflammatory bowel disease has been given equal weighting.

Finally, the story now presented is a culmination of 39 years of personal clinical experience and laboratory research in this field. This entailed attendance at many conferences and interaction with many colleagues. Events currently recorded are in the published literature and listed at the end of each chapter. The analytical outcomes now put forward may lack the punch of 'modern scientific journalism' demonstrated in commissioned work of leading scientific journals but rather provides an evolving theme. In this regard I apologise to anyone who may feel their field of work neglected. Causation at all times was central to the current narrative.

W.E.W.R.

Introduction

Bacteria, bacterial metabolism and bacterial metabolites in the gastrointestinal tract, more particularly the colon, have received modest scientific attention. An exception to this is the recent swell of genetic analyses of colonic bacteria now encapsulated in the term 'microbiome'. New definitions have arisen and the galaxy of bacteria found in any one human is referred to as an 'enterotype'. Pure microbiologists and environmental microbiologists have rarely aligned themselves with clinical microbiologists who study harmful bacteria that cause diseases. The daunting task is where to commence an analysis of colonic bacteria and even more pointedly how to locate harmful bacteria.

Bacterial metabolites have received a poor press. Sherwood Gorbach in 1976 nominated short chain fatty acids (also known as organic acids) in the colon as being harmful, a view then supported by many. Since that view was put, the opposite has been found to be true to the degree that the metabolic welfare of colonic epithelial cells is determined by these bacterial metabolites, thereby providing a starting plan for the search for the causation of ulcerative colitis.

Bacterial metabolism in a broad sweep includes the processing by bacteria of oxygen (O_2), nitrogen (N_2) carbon (C), hydrogen (H) and sulphur (S). A supply of each element is essential for bacteria in their metabolism. The effect of oxygen, the need for carbon and the production and disposal of hydrogen have found a niche in colonic bacterial metabolism. With regard to sulphur the microbiologist Sir John Postgate FRS believed sulphate-reducing bacteria unlikely to be found in the human colon, yet careful search has indicated a strong role for sulphate-reducing bacteria in the colon.

In the past, concern with nitrogen metabolism in the human colon centred on the production of carcinogenic nitrosamines. This view has relegated all consideration of nitrogen to be useful in colonic bacterial metabolism. Anaerobic bacterial metabolism as it occurs in the colon requires nitrogen. The colonic bacteria are an integral part of the 'global nitrogen' cycle, playing both a part in conservation of nitrogen as a usable substrate as well as in the loss of nitrogen as gaseous nitric oxide or nitrogen gas. Environmental and soil microbiologists have long grappled with the processing of nitrogen in soils and the biosphere. Nitrogen is invaluable for food production and the nutrition of the growing world population. The intermediary products of nitrogen metabolism, that is of the denitrification process, have strong effects on colonic function, particularly absorption. The products of bacterial nitrogen metabolism have been another stimulus to finding the causation of ulcerative colitis. The concept of nitroso-burn from excessive denitrification is well known in soil biochemistry and equally has currency in colonic epithelial metabolism where it causes damage.

Bacteria have been implicated in the causation of inflammatory bowel disease, not only of ulcerative colitis but more frequently of Crohn's disease. Formation of tissue granulomata in Crohn's disease has been the signpost to seek organisms that induce granuloma formation. Tuberculosis *(Mycobacteria pneumonia)* produces abundant granulomata in the lung, but a search amongst mycobacteria in tissues other than the lung has not produced any strong leads, but much controversy. The chemical agent 'lipopeptide' by which granulomata are induced in laboratory animals may also be derived from bacteria known as *Mycoplasma. Mycoplasma* were first associated with pneumonia in young people in 1944 by Eaton, and was thereafter referred to as Eaton's agent. *Mycoplasma pneumonia* was only identified 21 years later, but even then certainty was not accredited. Mycoplasmology emerged between 1950 and 1975, and more species are still being found today. Amongst *Mycoplasma* are species for which a disease has not yet been found.

Each chapter of this book is headed by a non-technical 'outline' to facilitate understanding of the chain of thoughts of the more technical sections of some chapters. These require a basic understanding of biology. Many chapters are less technical and complex than others.

W.E.W. Roediger
Adelaide, 2016

PART ONE

Ways and Means

–1–

Final conclusions about the causative factors of ulcerative colitis and Crohn's disease

OUTLINE: A most likely causative factor of ulcerative colitis is production of bacterial metabolites which in turn depends on dietary factors and the presence of bacteria that undergo 'denitrification'. Therapeutic modulation of diet and bacteria with resultant improvement of colitis lends support to these proposals. Crohn's disease is most likely associated with pathogenic *Mycoplasma fermentans*. The criteria that determine association as causation are tabulated. Evidence given in the book indicates that association of events in Crohn's disease and ulcerative colitis tentatively can be given a verdict of causation.

In compiling *Causative Factors of Ulcerative Colitis and Crohn's Disease* the hope was to replace, for the patient, distressing treatment processes, both medical and surgical, with better treatment options through a scientific understanding of the origin of ulcerative colitis and Crohn's disease. The philosophy encompassing personal research methodology was simple: positive leads in experimental research were worthwhile pursuing and negative results left as noted but not further evaluated. The aim always was to investigate human ulcerative colitis, not the colitis of mice or colitis of rats though a watchful eye was kept on developments in animal work. It is possible – and there are some examples – that clues for a disease process may emerge from animal research work.

In summary: for ulcerative colitis the initiating factors found were excessive bacterial production of nitric oxide with sulphide (see Chapter 7) by as yet undefined groups of bacteria in association with poor capacity for nitric oxide detoxification by the lining epithelial cells of the colon. The resultant breakdown of barrier function of the epithelial cells leads to elevation of immune cell activity beyond that normally present. Thus bacterial metabolites probably initiate and partially propagate ulcerative colitis, which is a disease of nitrosative stress. The therapeutic implications of these findings are given in Chapter 10.

For Crohn's disease the most likely bacterial association is *Mycoplasma fermentans* (see Chapter 16) which has a short initial invasive stage of tissue followed by a prolonged antigenic phase in tissues with resultant deep ulceration and fissuring. The organism may be found in the oral cavity and becomes pathogenic anywhere along the gastrointestinal tract. The therapeutic implications and stages of treatment are given in Chapter 17.

In general, with regard to bacterial metabolites (ulcerative colitis) and specific bacteria (Crohn's disease) Sir Austin Hill has questioned whether any association that is proposed may reflect causation.[1] Elevating an association to causation requires several attributes which are outlined in Table 1.1. Strength of association, specificity and temporality of association are important as well as biological gradient and plausibility. Aspects of these have been discussed throughout the chapters and a tentative case made that association of events from experiments may give a verdict of causation.

Table 1.1 Criteria that determine association or causation[1]

1. Strength of association
2. Consistency and unbiasedness of association
3. Specificity of the association
4. Temporality
5. Biological gradicnt
6. Biological plausibility
7. Coherence with previous knowledge
8. Experimental evidence
9. Reasoning by analogy

Hopefully knowledge of inflammatory bowel disease will be strengthened and become reliable through reproducibility of experimental results by experienced researchers and avoid non-reproducibility through poor scientific practice. Evolution of science is continual. For example, chemistry gave rise to chemical physiology, which in turn led to biochemistry, which evolved into molecular biology. Each of these categories brought new sophistications to experimental work. This is an example of scientific evolution. Currently Mycoplasma detection is signposted by the World Health Organisation as necessary in attempting to standardize assays for detection of mycoplasma-DNA.[2] These standards may in future be applied to analysis of tissue from Crohn's disease. In genetics, DNA sequencing of whole populations, such as Iceland,[3] may bring better analysis of variant genes for inflammatory bowel disease. With future developments 'hierarchies of evidence'[4] may emerge for the causation of ulcerative colitis and Crohn's disease and perhaps confirm or reject what has been proposed for disease causation in this book.

Ignorance has been a powerful drive for research.[5] The philosopher-scientist Erwin Schrödinger remarked that in an honest search for knowledge one has to tolerate ignorance for an indefinite period.[6] To this advice should be added that prejudging outcomes must be avoided. Measurement of outcomes needs to be unfettered, honest and embedded in clinical observations as much as possible. Clinical investigators are an imperilled species and experimental work should run in parallel with clinical observations. This approach has been followed in the formulation of this book.

References

1. Hill AB. The environment and disease: association or causation? Proc R. Soc Med 58:295–300 (1965)
2. Nubling CM, Baylis SA, Hanschmann KM et al. World Health Organization International standard to harmonize assays for detection of mycoplasma DNA. Appl Environ Microbiol. June (2015) in press
3. Editorial. Letters from Iceland. Nature Genetics 47:425 (2015)
4. Rawlins M. *Detestimonio*: on the evidence for decisions about the use of therapeutic interventions. Lancet 372:2152–2161 (2008)
5. Firestein S. Ignorance. How it drives science. Oxford University Press, New York (2012)
6. Schrödinger E. Nature and the Greeks; and Science and Humanism. Cambridge University Press, Cambridge (1996)

-2-

The impetus and history of ulcerative colitis and Crohn's disease

OUTLINE: Both ulcerative colitis and Crohn's disease have medically been categorized for just over 100 years. Various kinds of bacteria cause diarrhoea but are not known to produce ulcerative colitis or Crohn's disease. Separation of ulcerative colitis from Crohn's colitis was first recognized in 1960.

The causation of Crohn's disease and ulcerative colitis, the main categories of diseases listed as 'inflammatory bowel diseases' is, according to many experts, unknown.[1,2,3,4] Little commentary in the textbooks is devoted to explaining the causative processes that have engaged the minds of clinicians who have dedicated their work to ulcerative colitis and Crohn's disease. The prime benefit in bringing an approximation to the causes would be a better direction than the unknown, in the management of cases affected either with Crohn's disease or ulcerative colitis. Chronicity of the diseases has added greatly to the altered quality of life which also would be deserving of more research.

Ulcerative colitis

What medical heritage can be attributed to ulcerative colitis? Understanding bacillary dysentery around 1910, an era which was at a high point of microbiological discoveries, contracted to such specific organisms as *Shigella* species, *V. cholerae* and enteropathogenic *E. coli*.[5,6] The first isolate of *Shigella flexneri* in the Medical Collection UK was made in 1915[7]. Once diagnostic tests for these gut infections were refined it became possible to define a colitis, with ulcers or without, which could be chronic and associated with blood loss but for which no causative organism could be found. Idiopathic ulcerative colitis was identified as a distinct entity by 1895[8] but it was only with the use of the 'electric sigmoidoscope' by 1907[9] that the disease process along the colon could be confirmed. Past experts who had considered the history of ulcerative colitis, such as J. Kirsner and J. Goligher, concluded that 'in all probability we shall never know for certain who first described ulcerative colitis'.[10] The disease could only be defined after microbiological evaluation, direct mucosal visualisation and biopsy analysis. A personal guess is that wider recognition of ulcerative colitis occurred after 1910. The first ever recorded cases of paediatric ulcerative colitis were reported in 1923.[11]

While bloody diarrhoea and post mortem changes of ulcerative colitis were observed up to 1910, no clear cut identity of ulcerative colitis, as now diagnosed, could then be made. Antiquity does reveal ample records of diabetes and heart failure because of their clear cut chronic symptoms. A diagnostic test, the urine taste test, for diabetes was even developed more than a thousand years ago but testing for ulcerative colitis could not be done in antiquity and we therefore lack a long past description of present day ulcerative colitis.

Crohn's disease

Crohn's disease in its 'living' manifestation of either bowel obstruction or peritonitis was first described by the Scottish surgeon J.K. Dalziel in 1913.[12] At operation he was able to visibly inspect the diseased bowel which hitherto, due to lack of diagnostic special tests, was not possible. Prior to Dalziel a number of individual post mortem cases could have been Crohn's disease as put forward by Blonski and colleagues in 2011.[13] Dalziel described the small bowel as 'rigid as an eel' approximating the transmural thickening observed in Crohn's disease since Dalziel's observation.

Similar findings to Dalziel but less extreme pathological changes in the bowel were described by B.B. Crohn and colleagues in 1932.[10,14] Crohn designated the findings as 'regional ileitis' but subsequently this has been simplified to 'Crohn's disease'. The separation in clinical-pathological terms, between Crohn's disease of the colon and ulcerative colitis of the colon was made by 1960 by the combined description of a pathologist, B. Morson and a St. Mark's surgeon H.E. Lockhart-Mummery.[15] Further descriptive refinements of Crohn's disease have since then been made mostly for the observation of the earliest visible lesions of Crohn's disease along the gastro-intestinal tract.

The clinical categorisation of Crohn's disease and ulcerative colitis as noted in 2015 is just over 100 years old. Historically we have only had a short time to focus on both diseases. Their relative infrequency has not led to great inroads into the study of causation of these diseases. The general methodology and means by which the causation could be approximated is outlined in the following chapters.

References

1. Inflammatory Bowel Diseases Eds. J Satsangi and LR Sutherland, Churchill Livingstone, London, (2003)
2. Kirsners Inflammatory Bowel Disease, 6th Edition, Eds: RB Sartor and WJ Sandborn, Saunders Edinburgh (2004)
3. Inflammatory Bowel Disease, Eds. S Targan, F Shanahan and LC Karp, Wiley-Blackwell, Chichester (2010)
4. Challenges in Inflammatory Bowel Disease, 2nd Edition, Eds. DP Jewell, NJ Mortensen, A Steinhart, J Pemberton and BF Warren, Blackwell Publishing, Oxford (2006)
5. Tapeworms, Lice and Prion. DI. Grove, Oxford University Press, Oxford, (2014)
6. Molecular Microbiology, Diagnostic Principles and Practice, 2nd Ed. Eds. DH Persing et al., ASM Press, Washington DC (2011)
7. Matheras, Baker KS et al., Bacillary dysentery from World War 1 and NCTCI the first bacterial isolate in the National Collection, BMJ 384:1720 (2014)
8. White WH, Colitis, Lancet 145:537–538 (1895)
9. Lockhart-Mummery JP., The Causes of colitis with special reference to its surgical treatment, Lancet 169: 1638–1643 (1907)
10. Kirsner JB. Historical aspects of inflammatory bowel disease, J. Clin. Gastroenterol 10:286–297 (1988)
11. Helmholz HF. Chronic ulcerative colitis in childhood, Am J. Dis Child 26:418–430 (1923)
12. Dalziel TK. Chronic interstitial enteritis Br. Med. Journal ii:, 1068–1070 (1913)
13. Crohn's Disease, Eds. GR. Lichtenstein and EJ. Scherl, Slack Inc. New Jersey, (2011)
14. Crohn B.B. Ginzburg L. and Oppenheimer GD. Regional ileitis: a pathologic and clinical entity, JAMA 99:1323–1329 (1932)
15. Lockhart-Mummery HE. and Morson BC. Crohn's disease (regional enteritis of the large intestine) and its distinction from ulcerative colitis, GUT 1: 87–105 (1960)

-3-

The evolving philosophy of science and research of disease causation

OUTLINE: Greek science did not permit changeability and lacked human anatomical studies. European science in the 17th and 18th century evolved by quantitative methods of experimentation. Proposing a hypothesis was a guide to research but had many weaknesses. By questioning and answering with consequent model building, another method of scientific progression was possible. Criteria for causation of disease processes are given.

Even though the clinical picture of ulcerative colitis and Crohn's disease emerged one hundred years ago, the arduous path of the philosophy of science that preceded those 100 years brought varying emphasis on the scientific process that could be employed in experiments. In short the methodology with which causation of disease could be studied would vary with the development of the philosophy of science.

Greek science

The Ancient Greek or Hellenic culture of medicine was based in Miletus, Athens and Alexandria from where a peak of Greek medicine was reached in the 2nd century AD reflected in Galen's 20 volumes of written medical work.[1] The preceding Greek philosophy emphasised immutability. Apparent change was considered an illusion. The world consisted of four elements: earth, water, air and fire a concept that dominated 'science' thinking for 1000 years. The nature of matter was of a large number of elements described as seed theory or as refined by Aristotle 'the atomic theory'. From here science proceeded into the geometrization of nature and mathematical physics which under Archimedes became dominant. The move into biological research and zoology occurred under Hippocrates and Plato where zoological classification but not human anatomy were the mainstay. Helenistic philosophy did not permit exploration of human anatomy or biological evaluation by numbers because the concept of immutability and incontrovertible premises dominated.

Early European science

The first encouragement of mathematical analysis in a biological field was proposed by Roger Bacon, an Oxford monk, in 1267.[2] He also proposed that induction (the process of inferring principles from the observation of particular instances) be based on rigorous observation. His zeal emanated from a realization that the Christian calendar then used had errors which needed correction by observation and mathematical calculation. Bacon's exhortation waited 300 years to be applied to science, but during this interval great studies of human anatomy by Vesalius[3] and Fabricius in Italy were carried out and published.

In 1620 Francis Bacon, unrelated to his earlier namesake, who was a philosopher, thinker, political wheeler dealer and time server wrote *The New Organon*[4] which eschewed Greek immutability and proposed a new scientific method in which observation and experimentation were a prerequisite for the construction of scientific theory. Francis Bacon however did not include mathematical analyses in his suggestions. Bacon in his book provides several examples of the process of research current at his time of writing. Bacon's method was mindful of the close relationship of experimental practice and methodological processing of results. Bacon also defined the impediments of scientific method as 'idols and illusion' of existing thought, an exhortation as applicable in the 21st century as it was in 1625. Francis Bacon's books subsequently provided a backdrop to the founding of the Royal Society constituted in 1660.

Baconian principles of science and the newly described anatomy of humans were successfully brought together by William Harvey when he defined the heart as a pump. Centuries later it required the discovery of natural science, the 'living microcosm' in the Victorian era (1830–1902) and thereafter progression onto chemical analysis of tissue and cell preparations to provide a backdrop into the 20th century of human experimentation. The stage of modern experimental approach was set but with restrictions.

Later European science

The sway of 'the hypothesis'

The Baconian era set the dawn of the concept of 'hypothesis' which initially in 1596 was defined as 'a proposition or principle put forward or stated merely as a basis for reasoning or argument'. This definition has undergone much modification and philosophical analyses especially in the 20th century. Beveridge[5] in *The Art of Scientific Investigation* discusses the centrality of hypothesis to promoting the physical work of experimentation. Most hypotheses recorded by Beveridge proved to be wrong and caution was given not to cling to ideas proven useless. Beveridge also mentions that hypotheses may be used to introduce bias and filter data. If a hypothesis held good under all circumstances then it may be elevated to a category of theory.

The Austrian philosopher of science, Karl Popper writing from Europe and the UK[6] reasoned that the process of induction or deduction from a hypothesis can only be made by falsification and not verification of data. The proof of a hypothesis rests on defining where it does not apply. This concept has proved difficult to follow in modern scientific research but nevertheless drew attention to hypotheses as a potential weak link to research.

The concept of hypotheses found detractors especially in Isaac Newton and the philosopher David Hume. Newton put forward the primacy of experimentation, without a hypothesis, to construct a rule as to how reality operated. Hume introduced radical scepticism in saying one could not use past experiences in science to predict the future. However the concept of 'uniformity of nature' is put forward as a counter to the proposal of scepticism.

In human research the 'hypothesis' provides an inadequate approach as falsification and verification give incomplete answers. Glass and Hall[7] have proposed that 'the hypothesis' should be abandoned in favour of either a question or if sufficient data are available a model. It is better to see science as a quest for good questions to be answered rather than a bold hypothesis to refute.

There are many facets to the scientific process such as reality, rationality, imagination, initiation and simplicity. Ockham, an English monk, seven hundred years ago proffered the principle that we should apply simpler explanations when trying to account for observed facts. Included under 'reality' is that study or questions concerning humans far outweigh observations made in animal species. While results thus gained in humans may guide they cannot completely replace all the criteria for causation of disease as proposed by Evans[8] (Table 2.1). Finding causation of disease is a long exploratory journey.

Table 2.1 The modified Evans criteria for causation of disease[8]
1. Prevalence of disease and exposure to putative cause must match
2. Exposure to potential cause should be more common in those with disease
3. Spectrum of host responses should follow putative agent
4. A measurable host response to exposure to putative agents should regularly appear
5. Elimination or modification of putative cause should decrease incidence of disease
6. Biological and epidemiological sense should prevail in all criteria

In summary, studying patients in health and with inflammatory bowel disease, asking the right questions, doing the experiments, gaining reliable results, simplicity and modelling responses to fit causation was an approach taken in my personal research and in research quoted from others, as elucidated in the chapters that follow.

References

1. Freely J. The Flame of Miletus, IB Tauris (London) (2012)
2. Clegg B. The First Scientist, A Life of Roger Bacon, Constable (London) (2003)
3. Vesalius A. The Fabric of the Human Body: an annotated translation of the 1543 and 1555 Editions of De Humani Corporis Fabrica Libri Septem, Eds. D. Garrison and M. Hast, Karger (2014)
4. Bacon F. The New Organon, Edited by L. Jardine and M. Silverthorne, Cambridge University Press, Cambridge (2000)
5. Beveridge W I B, The Art of Scientific Investigation, Heinemann, London (1950)
6. Popper KR. The Logic of Scientific Discovery, Third impression, Hutchinson London (1962)
7. Glass DJ. and Hall N. A Brief History of the Hypothesis, Cell 134:378–381 (2008)
8. Evans AS. Causation and Disease, A Chronological Journey. Plenum Medical Book Company, New York (1993)

PART TWO

Ulcerative Colitis

-4-

The biological compartments of the colon: concepts in man or animal?

OUTLINE: Three compartments of the gut: bowel contents, lining cells and underlying immune cells were suitable for research of ulcerative colitis. Lining cells were chosen and four questions asked: what are their nutrients in health, how are these used in ulcerative colitis, could any metabolic abnormalities be reproduced by agents and would their elimination be of therapeutic value?

The intestinal tract from the oesophagus to rectum in transection comprises three distinct compartments most important in the study of inflammatory bowel disease.

1. The luminal contents in each section of the bowel
2. The lining cells or epithelial cells of the mucosa
3. The layer of immune cells deep to the surface epithelial cells, referred to as lamina propria

These three layers are enclosed by muscular layers both circular and longitudinal, through which a localised network of nerves traverse with outside connections to the central nervous system.

A search for the causation of ulcerative colitis would need to focus on one or all of the three biological compartments that is food in the small intestine and the microbial mass in the colon, the lining epithelial cells and mucosal immune system.

In the colon the number of 'cell' varieties for microbes is 600+ species, for the immune cells 10–20 different types and for colonic epithelial cells 1–5 related types. Based on chemical complexity, values for the number of chemical reactions in each of these three systems lie in the proportion of 1000:10:1 – the chemical diversity is greatest in the microbial mass and least in epithelial cells.[1] The chance of finding a metabolic abnormality is least in the microbial mass and easiest in the least complex system, the lining epithelial cells. Statistical argument[1] for study of the simplest systems was strong but mindful of the other two biological compartments and the potential interactions with epithelial cells.

In general the three compartments of the intestinal tract have attracted the interests of microbiologists, geneticists, biochemists and immunologists. A major consideration in their experimental work is whether the research is undertaken in animals or humans. Taking observations made in humans to animals often provides guidance of further research activity whereas using primarily animals and applying observations of these to humans is often fraught with great difficulty. The predictive value of animal research is extremely poor for human disease.[2] By and large animal models have not been tested for their validity or generalised ability to the human condition. Mouse models are extensively used in gastroenterological research.[3] As editorialized in *Nature Medicine* 'mice do not reproduce the patterns of gene expression induced by human inflammatory disease and this requires renewed discussion of the validity of animal models in translational research'[4]. Likewise colitis in rats or mice is not equatable with human disease particularly when pursuing causation of a disease process.[5]

Of the three biological compartments choice fell on the lining epithelial cells for experimentation. In the colon no such study had been conducted in the past. After lengthy discussion with clinical colleagues and staff of the Metabolic Research Laboratory, Radcliffe Infirmary, Oxford several questions arose. The biochemistry of the lining epithelial cells could not be fitted into any hypothesis but a series of questions (Table 3.1) arose that needed answers and thereby a plan of action was formulated which took considerable time to complete.

Table 3.1 Questions guiding future research
1. What were the chief nutrients and to what degree were these sustaining colonocytes?
2. Were there any metabolic lesions in colonocytes of ulcerative colitis?
3. Could agents be found that accounted for the metabolic lesions of ulcerative colitis?
4. Would eliminating the causative agent of any metabolic lesion add to the treatment of ulcerative colitis?

The above questions required investigation and research was conducted with human colonic epithelial cells to facilitate answers.

References

1. Roediger WEW. What sequence of pathogenetic events leads to acute ulcerative colitis? Disease Colon Rectum 31:482–487 (1988)
2. Bracken MB. Risk, Chance and Causation. Investigating the Origins and Treatment of Disease pp. 178–179. Yale University Press, New Haven (2013)
3. Low MJ. Mouse models in Gastroenterology research. Gastroenterology 143: 1410–1412 (2012)
4. Editorial. Of men, not mice. Nature Medicine 19:379 (2013)
5. Seok J, Warren HS, Cuenca AG. et al. Genomic responses in mouse models poorly mimic human inflammatory disease. PNAS 110:3507–3012 (2013)

-5-

Nutrient sustenance of colonic epithelial cells (colonocytes)

OUTLINE: Nutrition of the lining cells of the small bowel is 50% from ingested protein (glutamine) and 50% from amino acids (glutamine) released into the circulation from muscle. Lining cells of the large bowel are exclusively nourished from bacterial products: 70% of their metabolism is from a conjoined vinegar molecule known as butyrate, produced by bacterial fermentation. A reserve nutrient supply to colonic epithelial cells is not available from the circulation. Glucose is not metabolized to CO_2 by lining cells of either small or large bowel.

Experiments with colonic epithelial cells now termed 'colonocytes' needed a 'clean catch' system of these cells. Historically biochemical analyses of mammalian colonic tissue were done with mucosal scrapings or tissue slices. In the 1920's, mucosal scrapings of the colonic mucosa revealed that most of the glucose incubated with cell scrapings was converted to lactate and not oxidised to CO_2. This observation was then thought to be due to damage of colonic epithelial cells.[1] Subsequent biochemical experiments progressed to 'tissue slices' employed particularly with liver tissue that became the centre point of biochemical research. A giant leap forward occurred in the 1970s with the preparation of suspensions of isolated liver cells called 'hepatocytes', after in vivo perfusion of the liver with a chelating agent EDTA and hyaluronidase that broke down the tight epithelial junctions between cells. Isolated hepatocytes suspensions permitted multiple synchronous biochemical experiments that had good reproducibility.

Preparing isolated epithelial cells of the intestine seemed desirable if only to have an actual 'clean catch' system to undertake multiple experiments. The path was led by Watford and Lund in 1977.[2] Filling the lumen of the small bowel of the rat with the chelating agent EDTA to break down the tight epithelial junctions permitted collection of suspensions of epithelial cells that is 'enterocytes' for biochemical incubation with numerous nutrient solutions.[2] Watford was fortunate that he could rely on observations of his predecessors. Neptune in Taiwan[3] and Windmueller and Spaeth in the USA[4] had shown that glutamine was a substantial fuel for mucosal rings or perfused small intestine. This was subsequently confirmed by Watford et al. for isolated enterocytes of the small intestine of the rat.[2] The contribution of glutamine for enterocytes was from two sources, either luminal nutrient or nutrient release from muscle stores into the circulation particularly during starvation. The small intestine thus received protection by a guaranteed nutrient supply from muscle during starvation and thereby maintained optimal absorption from the small intestine whenever needed. Isolated enterocytes also revealed that most glucose in incubation media was converted to lactate and not oxidized to CO_2. Lactate absorbed into the portal system would again be converted to glucose in the liver. The benefits of isolating epithelial cells in the small intestine provided a guiding light and prompted isolation of epithelial cells from the colon.

The first preparation of viable and isolated colonic epithelial cells was achieved in 1979[1] in the Metabolic Research Laboratory of the Radcliffe Infirmary Oxford, then under the leadership of Sir Hans Krebs. In animals the whole rat colon was everted and incubated in an EDTA/ albumen solution and thereafter freed by gentle mechanical agitation which provided a good harvest of cells (Fig. 5.1) For human tissue mucosal strips from operative specimens were lifted by sharp dissection from the underlying muscle layers. Strips incubated with EDTA/hyaluronidase gave good harvest of human cells. A colonic tissue system was ready for biochemical analysis which previously was not possible.

Analyses of the nutrition of isolated colonocytes would include glucose and glutamine based on the results with enterocytes of small bowel (Fig. 5.2). Another potential fuel of the gut lining emerged from research work on fermentative organs such as the rumen of cattle and kangaroos as well as the colon of rabbits. Kiddle et al.[5] in 1951 revealed that butyrate was taken up in the rumen wall but very little butyrate was found in the blood leaving the rumen. Thereafter Professor Frank Hird at Melbourne University, Melbourne, showed with Susan Henning that another fermentative organ, the colon of the rabbit, converted butyrate to

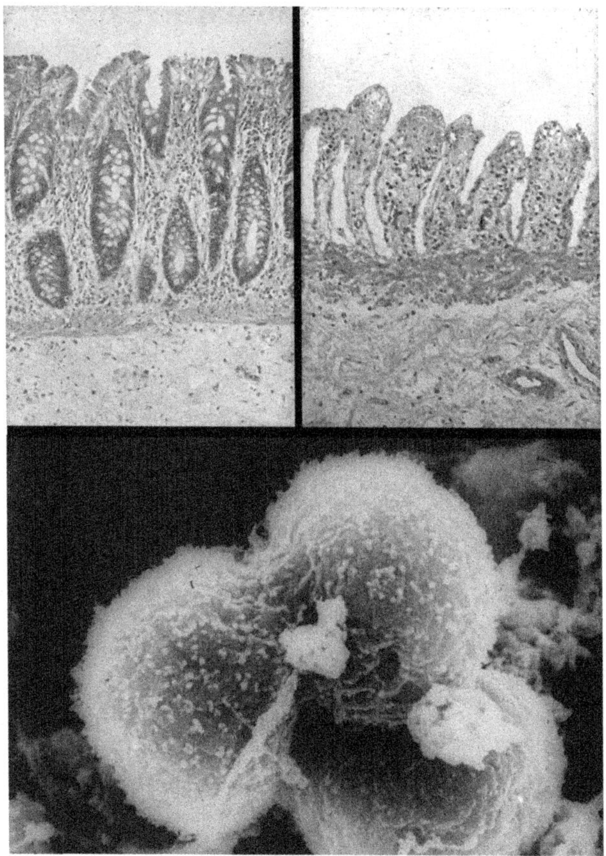

Figure 5.1 Human colonic mucosa in health before and after removal of surface epithelial cells (colonocytes). All immune cells of the lamina propria are left intact. Below, isolated cells shown by scanning electron microscope.

CO_2 and ketone bodies.[6] Much of their subsequent work, all performed on Australian mammals focussed on ketogenesis and the purpose of the ketogenic reaction in fermentative organs.

An analysis with isolated colonocytes in human and rats therefore included glucose, glutamine, butyrate and ketone bodies measuring each separately and in conjunction with each other to establish the utility of

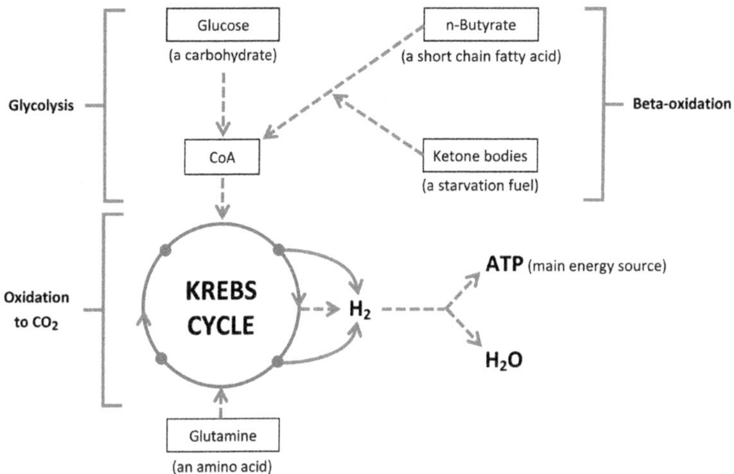

Figure 5.2 Nutrients involved in the metabolism and energy formation in colonocytes

these fuels. Water-bath manometry to measure oxygen consumption and the disappearance of substrates as well as radio-labelled measurement of CO_2 from labelled glucose, pyruvate, glutamine and butyrate followed. In summary the results were that the preferential fuels were butyrate > ketone bodies > glutamine > glucose.[7] Very little glucose was oxidized to CO_2. These observations first conducted in rats were replicated in isolated human colonocytes and showed that butyrate provided 70% of the oxidative cell energy.[8]

Of all the water soluble fatty acids with a carbon length from C_2 to C_{14}, butyrate remains the premier fuel for colonocytes.[9] Butyrate in colonocytes is also the basic building block for lipid synthesis[10] providing the basis of structural lipids for organelles and cell membranes. A number of scientists have confirmed the primacy of butyrate as a metabolic fuel in colonocytes.[11, 12]

If butyrate is so prominent in colonic epithelial nutrition then function of the epithelial lining should be in parallel with the availability of luminal butyrate. Depriving the colonic mucosa of butyrate[13] severely impairs sodium absorption and converts absorption in the colon to secretion. The practical reality is that in human starvation where little butyrate would be formed in the colon severe diarrhoea would follow.[14] Every prisoner of war in WWII who had lost more than 20% of body weight had severe diarrhoea.[15]

Colonocytes from germ free animals where luminal butyrate is deficient show decreased oxidative phosphorylation and 'ATP' formation establishing a condition of 'energy deficiency'.[16] This deficiency can be converted back to normal by supply or exogenous butyrate to isolated colonocytes prepared from germ free rats.

The nutrient profile of colonocytes revealed a strong dependence for all oxidation and lipid synthesis as well as epithelial function on a product of bacteria, that is n-butyrate. Anaerobic bacteria therefore predominantly sustain colonocytes and in the absence of n-butyrate no fall-back fuel, such as the dual sided supply of glutamine for enterocytes, is available for colonocytes. Neither glucose, ketones or glutamine could make up for the loss of bacterially produced n-butyrate. With this information the stage was set for studying fuel utilization in disease, that is ulcerative colitis.

References

1. Roediger WEW, Truelove SC. Method of preparing isolated colonic epithelial cells (colonocytes) for metabolic studies. GUT 20:484–488 (1979)
2. Watford MM., Lund P, Krebs HA. Isolation and metabolic characteristics of rat and chicken enterocytes. Biochem J. 178:589–596 (1979)
3. Neptune EM, Respiration and oxidation of various substrates by ileum in vitro. Am. J Physiol. 329–332 (1965)
4. Windmueller HG and Spaeth AE. Identification of ketone bodies and glutamine as the major respiratory fuels in vivo for post absorptive rat small intestine. J. Biol.Chem. 253:69–76 (1978)
5. Kiddle P, Marshall RA, Philipson AT. A comparison of the mixtures of acetic, propionic and butyric acids in the rumen and in the blood leaving the lumen. J. Physiol. 113:207–217 (1951)
6. Henning SJ and Hird FJR, Ketogenesis from butyrate and acetate by the caecum and the colon of rabbits. Biochem J. 130:785–790 (1972)
7. Roediger WEW. Utilization of nutrients by epithelial cells of the colon. Gastroenterology 83:424–429 (1982)
8. Roediger WEW. Role of anaerobic bacteria in the metabolic welfare of the colonic mucosa in man. GUT 21:793–798 (1980)
9. Roediger WEW, Nance S. Selective reduction of fatty acid oxidation in colonocytes: correlation with ulcerative colitis. Lipids 25:646–652 (1990)
10. Roediger WEW, Kapaniris O, Millard S. Lipogenesis from n-butyrate in colonocytes. Mol. Cell Biochem. 118:113–118 (1992)
11. Ardawi MSM, Newsholme EA. Fuel utilization in colonocytes of the rat. Biochem. J. 231:713–719 (1985)
12. Fleming SE, Fitch MD, Devries S et al. Nutrient utilization by cells isolated from rat jejunum, caecum and colon. J. Nutrition 121:869–878 (1991)

13. Roediger WEW, Rae DA. Trophic effect of short chain fatty acids on mucosal handling of ions by the defunctioned colon. Br.J.Surg. 69:23–25 (1982)
14. Roediger WEW. The starved colon – diminished mucosal nutrition, diminished absorption and colitis. Dis Colon Rectum 33:858–862 (1990)
15. Thaysen EH, Thaysen JH. Hunger diarrhoea. Acta Med. Scand Suppl. 274:124–160 (1952)
16. Donohoe DR, Wali A, Brylawski BP et al. Microbial regulation of glucose metabolism and cell-cycle progression in mammalian colonocytes. PLOS One 7:1–9 (2012)

-6-

The biochemical lesions in colonocytes of ulcerative colitis

OUTLINE: Lining cells in ulcerative colitis are unable to use butyrate for nutrition and increasingly use less efficient glucose. The biochemical currency of cell energy, co-enzyme A (CoA) is reduced in colitis. Production of fat in colonocytes for their assembly of membranes, production of cell proteins for bonding together colonocytes and production of mucus for cell protection are all reduced in ulcerative colitis. These changes are summated in the term 'energy deficiency disease' and constitute 'biochemical lesions'.

The concept of a biochemical lesion was first described in 1931[1] and more fully explained by its originator, Sir Rudolph Peters of Cambridge University, in 1969.[2] In essence the biochemical lesions are biochemical derangements either in organs or cells, that can strongly be associated with a disease process. Observations could be taken from actively metabolizing cells or changes observed with the light/electron microscope and taken to reflect metabolic alteration.

With the preferred nutrients of colonocytes established and the dependency of colonic function on the preferred fuel n-butyrate also established, it became possible to explore the nutritional profile in ulcerative colitis with the self same nutrients used in health. Wherever possible the severity of colitis, whether quiescent, moderately severe or acute, was correlated with the metabolic profile of colonocytes prepared from the colitic colon.

A summary of the biochemical lesions found in ulcerative colitis (and also some in Crohn's disease) are given as outlined below. Each is described in more detail in the subsequent paragraphs.

1. There is a failure of butyrate oxidation with a compensatory switch to glucose oxidation in colonocytes of ulcerative colitis.
2. There is a significant lowering of measurable free CoA in the colonic mucosa of ulcerative colitis and Crohn's disease.
3. There is a failure in ulcerative colitis of lipid cell-membrane folding and tight junction alignment compared to healthy colonocytes.
4. There is diminished capacity of detoxification in ulcerative colitis particularly of phenol as well as reduced detoxification of reactive nitrogen by glutathione in colonocytes.
5. There is a failure of mucus synthesis by colonocytes in ulcerative colitis.

1. Failed butyrate oxidation

Impairment of butyrate oxidation in colonocytes of ulcerative colitis was originally observed by measuring overall oxygen consumption and the contribution made to oxygen consumption by butyrate and glucose in quiescent, active and severe colitis.[(3)] Impairment of butyrate oxidation was found in all forms of ulcerative colitis and subsequently confirmed by using rectal biopsies.[(4)] Three subsequent studies conducted *in vivo* confirmed impaired butyrate oxidation. By measuring the contribution of butyrate to rectal-bicarbonate generation,[(5)] $^{14}CO_2$ generation in vivo[(6)] and $^{13}CO_2$ generation in labelled expired air[(7)] after rectal installation of labelled butyrate. Study of a large number of patients again confirmed the impairment of butyrate oxidation in ulcerative colitis.[(8)] Enhanced glycolysis, as was originally found,[(3)] was subseq uently found in the colonic mucosa by positron emission tomography scanning[(9, 10)] of fluorine labelled glucose. These positive scans have been attributed to both metabolism of colonocytes and activated immune cells and need further elucidation. Positive scans in colitis in remission[(11)] suggests an origin from colonocytes rather than activated immune cells for the enhanced glycolysis.

2. Lowered free CoA levels and colonocytes of ulcerative colitis

Coenzyme-A (CoA) is an essential intracellular molecule involved in cell energy production alternatively expressed as ATP. CoA is essential for the oxidation of butyrate and glucose. (See Fig. 5.2) Six times as much CoA is needed for the oxidation of butyrate than oxidation of glucose. Much of the research of CoA in colonocytes emanated from the Mayo Clinic and historically from the Johns Hopkins Hospital in Baltimore where haematologists and nutritionists undertook most of the research. The defining study of the colonic mucosa in 1976 revealed a lowered level of CoA in the colonic mucosa in ulcerative colitis and Crohn's disease.[12] This study revealed that CoA was inactivated or entrapped and not actually lost from the mucosa. The reason for this could not be established. In animals but not in man, CoA deficiency can be nutritionally induced by pantothenic acid deficiency.[13] In pigs creating a low level of mucosal CoA impairs electrolyte transport[14] and sets up a colitis similar to the distribution along the colon and histologic appearance of that of human ulcerative colitis.[13] The interest in pantothenic acid in humans has waned as no known deficiency has ever been found. The research work on pantothenic acid has consequently languished. An explanation of low CoA level in colitis was subsequently found (see Chapter 7).

3. Failure of colonocyte membrane and tight junction assembly in ulcerative colitis

Under the light microscope colonocytes in quiescent colitis appear normal like healthy, non-diseased colonocytes but with the transmission electron microscope and scanning electron microscope colonocytes in quiescent colitis show notable abnormalities.[15,16] The mild abnormalities found in quiescent colitis with the transmission electron microscope are accentuated in acute colitis as shown in numerous studies conducted in the 1960s and 1970s. Diminishment and distortion of the surface microvilli of colonocytes with vacuolisation of cell organelles were the most frequent changes observed.[17] Surface membrane changes of colonocytes would involve changes in lipid assembly or lipid availability, features often attributed to oxidative or nitrosative 'stress' to cells.

The scanning electron microscope of freeze-fractured colonocytes of ulcerative colitis showed diminished 'meshing' of tight junctions between colonocytes,[18,19] a structural domain that regulates mucosal permeability. Tight junctions are dependent on efficient protein synthesis in colonocytes of which several subtypes (occludins, claudin, cadherin, catenin) have been delineated.[20] Tight junctions are also dependent on a specific milieu particularly calcium which provides electrogenic qualities to the surface epithelium. The electrogenic qualities of the surface colonocytes are severely degraded in acute ulcerative colitis.[21]

Another finding on transmission electron microscopy in acute colitis is cell blebbing in colonocytes.[15,16] Cell blebbing has also been studied in another cell system, that is hepatocytes of the liver. In hepatocytes blebbing, which is reversible, is due to depletion of the energy currency ATP and diminished thiol groups most notably, glutathione.[22]

Of the above observations the lack of lipid synthesis for cell lining membranes, and diminishment in ATP were guiding features in order to define a precipitating cause for damage of colonocytes.

4. Failure of detoxification by colonocytes in ulcerative colitis

One of the major defences of colonocytes to the external environment is their capacity to detoxify injurious agents.[23] Colonocytes are analogous to and equally capable as liver cells in their ability to detoxify injurious agents. Most detoxification processes are dependent on specific enzyme activities and on a good supply of energy, most notably ATP.

The process of sulphation in colonocytes requires 'activated sulphate' and ATP together with enzymes in order to inactivate phenols or, more physiologically, to sulphate mucus[24] to stabilize mucus structure. Phenol detoxification in active ulcerative colitis, but not Crohn's disease, is severely impaired[24] which is another example of a 'biochemical lesion' in colonocytes of ulcerative colitis.

A further process of toxicant control is that effected by glutathione, usually implicated in oxidation – reduction control[25] but also involved in the detoxification of nitric oxide with a consequent production of nitrosothiols: that is nitric oxide reacts with the thiol group of glutathione. Both the quantity of glutathione[25] and the amount of reduced glutathione is altered in ulcerative colitis[26] suggesting either diminished synthesis or excessive consumption of glutathione. The latter is suggested by a significant increase of nitrosothiol groups in ulcerative colitis.[27] Transfer of toxic agents to glutathione is controlled by enzymes such as gluthathione transferase which have a noted genetic variation in ulcerative colitis[28] and certain of these enzyme patterns have been implicated in the genesis of ulcerative colitis.

5. Failure of mucus production by colonocytes

One of the diagnostic criteria on biopsies of the colonic mucosa in ulcerative colitis is depletion of mucus content in colonocytes affected by colitis [(29)]. Colonocytes are the prime producers of mucus the production of which is dependent on butyrate metabolism and which when inhibited by exogenous agents, also diminishes mucus production.[(30)] Reduced mucus production was confirmed by others[(31)] and sulphation of mucus found impaired in ulcerative colitis[(32)] in line with impaired sulphation found in the detoxifying processes. Changes of mucus subclasses or mucus fractions have also been found in ulcerative colitis.[(33)] Whether these changes are due to altered mucus synthesis as mentioned above or due to genetic changes associated with ulcerative colitis is not known.

Conclusion

A summation of the biochemical lesions as outlined in (1–5) above leads to the conclusion of an 'energy deficient disease'. Energy in biological systems can be expressed in several ways: as heat production or calories from food, as chemical energy such as ATP (activated phosphate) production, as consumption of oxygen, as mechanical work reflected as ergs or as electrical measurement such as millivolts on the surface of colonocytes. The prime deficiency in colonocytes of ulcerative colitis is a lowered ATP content[(34)] which leads to a multitude of changes in cell function and behaviour in colonocytes represented diagrammatically in Figure 6.1.

A search for the cause of 'energy deficiency' as seen in colonocytes of ulcerative colitis was made and is given in the next chapter.

References

1. Gavrilescu N, Peters RA. Biochemical lesions in vitamin B deficiency. Biochem. J. 25:1397–1409 (1931)
2. Peters RA. The biochemical lesion and its historical development. Br. Med. Bull. 25:223–226 (1969)
3. Roediger WE. The colonic epithelium in ulcerative colitis: an energy deficiency disease? Lancet 316: 712–715 (1980)
4. Chapman MAS, Grahn MF. Boyle MA. et al. Butyrate oxidation is impaired in the colonic mucosa of sufferers of quiescent ulcerative colitis. GUT 35:73–76 (1994)
5. Roediger WEW, Lawson MJ, Kwok V. et al. Colonic bicarbonate output as a test of disease activity in ulcerative colitis. J. Clin. Pathol. 37:704–707 (1984)
6. Den Hond E, Hiele M, Evenepoel P. et al. In vivo butyrate metabolism and colonic permeability in extensive ulcerative colitis. Gastroent. 115:584–590 (1998)

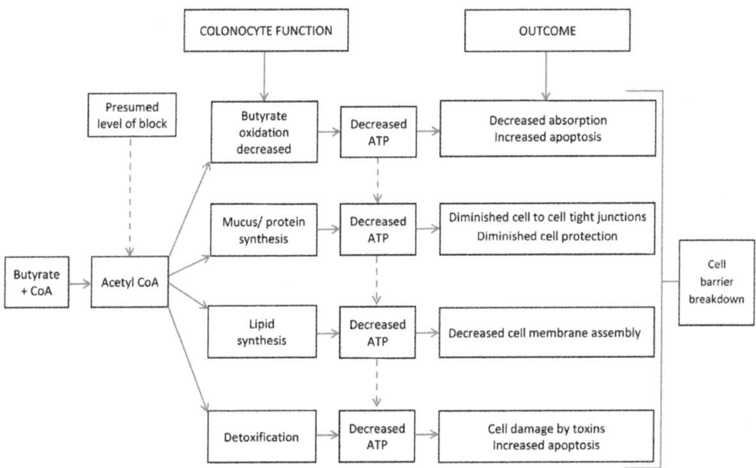

Figure 6.1 Features of the biochemical lesions in colonocytes of ulcerative colitis and the functional consequences.

7. Kato K, Ishii Y, Mizuno S. et al. Usefulness of rectally administering (1-^{13}C) – butyrate for breath test in patients with active and quiescent ulcerative colitis. Scand. J. Gastroent. 42:207–214 (2007)
8. De Preter V, Bulteel V, Suenaert P. et al. Pouchitis, similar to active ulcerative colitis, is associated with impaired butyrate oxidation by intestinal mucosa. Inflamm. Bowel Dis. 14:335–340 (2009)
9. Lemberg DA, Issenman RM, Cawdron R et al. Positron emission tomography in the investigation of pediatric inflammatory bowel disease. Inflamm. Bowel Dis. 11:733–738 (2005)
10. Meisner RS, Spier BJ, Einarsson S. et al. Pilot study using PET/CT as a novel, non-invasive assessment of disease activity in inflammatory bowel disease. Inflamm. Bowel Dis. 13:1993–1000 (2007)
11. Rubin DT, Surma BL, Gavzy SJ et al. Positron emission tomography. (PET) used to image sub clinical inflammation associated with ulcerative colitis (UC) in remission. Inflamm. Bowel Dis. 15:750–755 (2009)
12. Ellestad-Sayed JJ, Nelson RA, Adson MA et al. Pantothenic acid, coenzyme A and human chronic ulcerative and granulomatous colitis. Am.J.Clin. Nutr. 29:1333–1338 (1976)
13. Wintrobe MM, Follis RH, Alcayaga R. et al. Pantothenic acid deficiency in swine. Bull. Johns Hopkins Hosp. 73:313–340 (1943)
14. Nelson RA. Intestinal transport, coenzyme A and colitis in pantothenic acid deficiency. Am.J. Clin. Nutr. 21:495–501 (1968)
15. Delpre G, Avidor I, Steinherz R et al. Ultrastructural abnormalities in endoscopically and histologically normal and involved colon in ulcerative colitis. Am. J. Gastroent. 84:1038–1046 (1989)

16. Balazs M. and Kovacs A. Ulcerative colitis: electron microscopic studies with special reference to development of crypt abscesses. Dis. Colon Rectum 32:327–334 (1989)
17. Donnellan WL. Early histological changes in ulcerative colitis. Gastroent. 50:519–540 (1966)
18. Madara JL. Loosening tight junctions. Lessons from the intestine. J. Clin. Invest. 83:1089–1094 (1989)
19. Schmitz H. Barmeyer C, Fromm M et al. Altered tight junction structure contributes to the impaired epithelial barrier function in ulcerative colitis. Gastroent. 116:301–329 (1999)
20. Ivanov AI, Nusrat A and Arkos CA. The epithelium in inflammatory bowel disease: potential role of endocytosis of junctional proteins in barrier disruption. Novartis Foundation Symposium 263:115–132 (2004)
21. Edmonds CJ and Pilcher D. Electrical potential difference and sodium and potassium fluxes across rectal mucosa in ulcerative colitis. GUT 14:784–789 (1973)
22. Jewell SA, Bellomo G, Thor H et al. Bleb formation in hepatocytes during drug metabolism is caused by disturbances in thiol and calcium homeostasis. Science 217:1257–1259 (1982)
23. Roediger WE and Babidge W. Human colonocyte detoxification. Gut 41:731–734 (1997)
24. Ramakrishna BS, Roberts-Thomson IC, Pannall PR et al. Impaired sulphation of phenol by the colonic mucosa in quiescent and active ulcerative colitis. GUT 32:46–49 (1991)
25. Holmes EW, Yong SL, Eiznhamer D et al. Glutathione content of colonic mucosa: evidence for oxidative damage in active ulcerative colitis. Dig Dis Sci. 43:1088–1095 (1998)
26. Dido B, Hack V, Hochlehnert A et al. Impairment of intestinal glutathione synthesis in patients with inflammatory bowel disease. GUT 42:485–492 (1998)
27. Roediger WEW, Cummins A and Cowled P. Tissue nitrosothiol levels in acute ulcerative colitis – a step in disease induction. Nitric Oxide. Biol. Chem. 19:546 (2008)
28. Broekman MM, Bos C, Te Morsche RH et al. GST Theta null genotype is associated with an increased risk for ulcerative colitis. J. Hum.Genet. 59:575–580 (2014)
29. Smithson JE, Campbell A, Andrews JM et al. Altered expression of mucins throughout the colon in ulcerative colitis. GUT 40:234–240 (1997)
30. Finnie IA, Dwarakanath AD, Taylor BA et al. Colonic mucin synthesis is increased by sodium butyrate. GUT 36:93–99 (1995)
31. Cope GF, Heatley RV, Kelleher J. et al. In vitro mucus glycoprotein production by colonic tissue from patients with ulcerative colitis. GUT 29:229–234 (1988)
32. Raouf AH, Tsai HH, Parker N. et al. Sulphation of colonic and rectal mucin in inflammatory bowel disease: reduced sulphation of rectal mucus in ulcerative colitis. Clin. Sci 83;623–626 (1992)
33. Podolsky DK, Isselbacher KJ. Composition of human colonic mucin. Selective alteration in inflammatory bowel disease. J.Clin. Invest. 77:1263–1271 (1986)
34. Kameyama J, Narui H, Inui M. et al. Energy level in large intestinal mucosa in patients with ulcerative colitis. Tohoku J. Exp. Med. 143:253–4 (1984)

-7-

Agents causing the biochemical lesions in colonocytes of ulcerative colitis

OUTLINE: Reproduction of the biochemical lesions by agents was explored. The supply of butyrate and enzymes involved in butyrate oxidation are unimpaired in ulcerative colitis. Sulphide (SH) on its own was not damaging but sulphide with nitric oxide (NO) exactly reproduced the damage pattern seen in ulcerative colitis. Sulphide increases bacterial nitric oxide production forty-fold. The source of sulphides are a high protein (meat) intake and nitric oxide production related to a high nitrogen content of food. Certain denitrifying bacteria and other bacteria produce NO+SH. The, as yet unnamed, bacteria are perhaps more abundant in ulcerative colitis.

Confirmation from many directions which all showed a decrease of butyrate oxidation in colonocytes in parallel with the severity of ulcerative colitis, led to experimental probing with healthy colonocytes, as well as attempts by therapeutic innovation, to define the causation of the altered butyrate oxidation in ulcerative colitis. Few investigations gave consideration to the three major biochemical lesions, that is (1) decreased butyrate oxidation, (2) altered lipid synthesis and (3) a lowered CoA content in human colonocytes. The following is a series of explorations that were aimed at defining the origin of altered butyrate oxidation and to answer the question 'where-from the derivation of the biochemical lesion' in colonocytes of ulcerative colitis.

The list below reflects progressive scientific thinking over 10–15 years in an attempt to define the agents for the biochemical lesions in colonocytes of ulcerative colitis.

1. Lowered availability of luminal butyrate
2. Altered butyrate transport into colonocytes
3. Enzyme control of butyrate oxidation

4. Action of 'substituted' fatty acids
5. Luminal colonic sulphide
6. Nitrogen compounds in the colon: ammonia, nitrite, nitric oxide
7. Combined action of nitric oxide and sulphide

1. Lowered availability of luminal butyrate

Breuer et al.[1] and Scheppach et al.[2] in the early 1990's proposed an insufficiency of luminal butyrate to be causative of ulcerative colitis. They embarked on therapeutic trials of butyrate enemas to overcome the proposed deficiency. Results of their therapeutic trials revealed a slight improvement of proctitis which subsequently was difficult to reproduce.[3] Butyrate enemas are odoriferous and unpleasant to use and further studies have remained in abeyance. Measurements, furthermore, of luminal concentrations of butyrate in active ulcerative colitis have shown an excess rather than insufficiency of butyrate both in adults[4] and children.[5] A search for other explanations of impaired butyrate oxidation by colonocytes seemed necessary.

2. Altered butyrate transport into colonocytes

Butyrate and other short chain fatty acids are absorbed in the colon by non ionic diffusion and by active transport via a monocarboxylic acid transporter (MCT1). The proportionality of absorption due to each process has not been determined. The MCT1 transporter is located in the cell membrane of colonocytes. Thibault et al.[6,7] mainly but also others have suggested that diminished utilization of butyrate could be due to a transport deficiency of butyrate. Results of their work suggest that transport failure is secondary to inflammation and not a primary defect. Electron microscopical changes of cell membranes of colonocytes (Chapter 6) give support to such an interpretation.

3. Altered enzyme control of butyrate oxidation

The fatty acid oxidation pathway of butyrate, the enzymes involved in oxidation and additional metabolic features have been outlined in reference books and articles.[8,9] The enzyme controlling butyrate-CoA dehydrogenisation, butyrate-CoA dehydrogenase, was significantly increased in activity in the mucosa of ulcerative colitis.[9] A further enzyme, thiolase, which also brings butyrate to acetyl-CoA appeared lower in activity in acute ulcerative colitis.[9] A finding also confirmed by Santhanam et al.[10] in a separate study. A further conclusion of analyses of enzyme activity was that in ulcerative colitis in remission no substantial deficiency of enzyme activity controlling butyrate oxidation was found.[9] Altered gene expression of enzymes controlling fatty acid oxidation was however found in colonocytes of acute ulcerative colitis.[11] There appears agreement that a primary impairment of enzyme activity in colonocytes of ulcerative colitis could not be found and that enzyme changes in activity in acute ulcerative colitis were secondary to inflammation or inflammatory factors such as cytokines or possibly reactive oxygen/nitrogen species.[10]

4. Action of 'substituted' fatty acids

The three dominant short chain fatty acids, acetate, propionate and butyrate, in the colon are 2,3 and 4 carbon chain lengths of which the hydrogen groups may be substituted, the best known being a sulphydryl group. Such a substitution produces mercapto-acetate, mercapto-propionate and mercapto-butyrate. 3-Mercapto-propionate is a well established inhibitor of fatty acid oxidation in the heart[12] which led to a search of a similar action in colonocytes. All three mercapto fatty acids decreased oxidation of butyrate but did not enhance glucose oxidation.[13] Mercapto fatty acids are not found in abundance in the colonic lumen but mercapto-acetate is usually present.[14] Of the other substituted fatty acids bromobutyrate and bromo-octanoate reduced butyrate oxidation[13,15] and also caused colitis in experimental animals, however bromo fatty acids have not been reported in human faecal specimens. The place of mercapto fatty acids in the causation of the biochemical lesions of ulcerative colitis remains an open question.

5. Luminal colonic sulphide

Hydrogen sulphide in general is toxic to animal and human tissues thereby potentially being a causative agent of ulcerative colitis. Research at the Dunn School of Nutrition, Cambridge UK, under J. Cummings investigated, in terms of bacterial metabolism, the colonic fermentative formation/absorption of bacterial short chain fatty acids[16] and the disposal of bacterial hydrogen formed.[17] The bacterial formation of sulphide by sulphate reducing bacteria was also studied.[18] The Cambridge research team demonstrated that sulphate-reducing bacteria were more plentiful and more robust in the colon of ulcerative colitis patients than in control cases.[19] These observations were confirmed by others who found these bacteria more numerous in both acute and quiescent ulcerative colitis.[20] Surprisingly the level of hydrogen sulphide, despite high counts of sulphate reducing bacteria was not found to be elevated in ulcerative colitis[21] at least in a 'static' study where hydrogen sulphide production over 24 hours was not measured. Certainly hydrogen sulphide can be toxic to healthy human colonocytes[22] but only in very high concentrations and under conditions where substrates needed for detoxification of hydrogen sulphides by colonocytes were not provided in the cell incubation medium.

A role for hydrogen sulphide in the causation of ulcerative colitis cannot be completely negated. A high meat and protein intake in the diet has a propensity to elevate colonic sulphide levels[23] and a high meat intake frequently precedes an attack of acute ulcerative colitis.[24] Further indirect support for sulphide in the pathogenesis of ulcerative colitis comes from the observation with 5-amino salicylic acid (5-ASA), contained in salazopyrin, the most frequently used drug to ameliorate ulcerative colitis. Both 5-ASA and salazopyrin reduce the fermentative production of sulphide from sulphur amino acids when assessed in batch culture of colonic bacteria.[18, 25]

A final factor in the potential of hydrogen sulphide causing damage to colonocytes is the capacity of colonocytes to detoxify hydrogen sulphide. Detoxification to methanethiol[26] or the action of rhodanese[27] to produce thiocyanate are robust in healthy colonocytes but may wane in severe ulcerative colitis.[28] A co-factor for sulphide detoxification is cyanide, the chief source of which is cigarette smoke. Smokers, while smoking but not after cessation of smoking, are protected against the formation of ulcerative colitis,[29] perhaps by this mechanism.

The overall dilemma of the role of sulphide in the causation of ulcerative colitis is highlighted in a detailed review.[30] The key question that emerges from all investigations is whether sulphide is the main agent or a co-factor with other agents in bringing about ulcerative colitis. The answer will be considered in Section 7.

6. Nitrogen and nitroso compounds in the biochemical lesions of ulcerative colitis

Before focusing on the biochemical lesions due to nitrogen, some general remarks about nitrogen metabolism in the colon are needed. The chemical definition of nitroso compounds is that of compounds containing the monovalent radical –NO. These radicals form an integral part of the global nitrogen cycle[31] (Fig. 7.1) where inert nitrogen (N_2) in the atmosphere is converted to assimilable nitrogen in soils, sea water and human colon for use by bacteria and plants for growth. The human colon is part of the global nitrogen cycle where the oxides of nitrogen:nitrate (NO_3) nitrite (NO_2), nitric oxide (NO) and nitrous oxide (N_2O) reflect usable and assimilable forms of nitrogen which in its gaseous form, N_2, is metabolically inert.

Apart from bacterial growth, nitrogen also plays a central part in the respiration of bacteria in the colon, soils and deep sea water where an oxygen free (anaerobic) environment is maintained. Oxygen is nevertheless still required by colonic bacteria in their respiration for reduction of hydrogen to water. The oxides of nitrogen (NO_3, NO_2, NO, N_2O) provide this oxygen and these have, as shown since 1902, been known as essential for bacterial growth. A nitrate reduction test[32] was devised in the 1920s to assist the biochemical identification of bacteria which were classified as either being able or not able to reduce nitrate to nitrite.[33] It has now been established that oxides of nitrogen are reduced to nitrogen gas in a stepwise fashion, a process referred to as denitrification (Fig. 7.2).[34] Oxides of nitrogen may also be reduced to ammonia, a process referred to as assimilatory nitrogen reduction.[35] The first two agents in denitrification (NO_3 and NO_2) are solutes and the last three (NO, N_2O and N_2) are gases. Noteworthy is that in experiments, nitrite (NO_2) and nitric oxide (NO) are used interchangeably the respective 'forms' depending on pH, partial pressure and ionic content.

The entry of nitrate and nitrite into the colon of animals has been called into question. In the colon cleared of bacteria much nitrate/nitrite enters the colon transmucosally[36] but in the presence of bacteria nitrate and nitrite levels are barely measurable.[37,38] In humans considerable nitrate is found in ileal effluent and the content is increased by a nitrogen-rich diet.[39] Whether more nitrate enters the colon in ulcerative colitis than in health is not known.

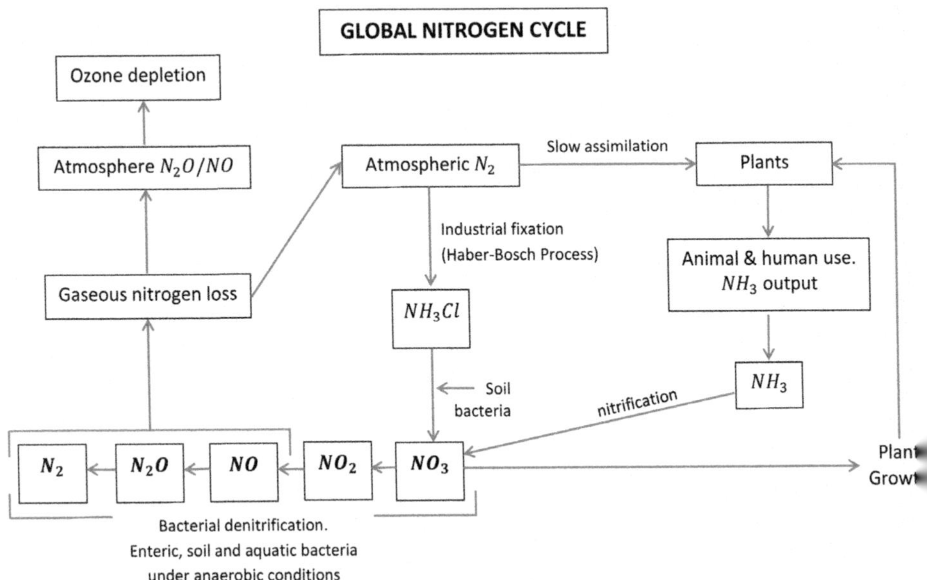

Figure 7.1 The nitrogen cycle between atmospheric nitrogen and nitrogen of animal, plant and bacterial metabolism, that is bacteria of the gut, soil and aquatic environments.

Measurement of nitrogen and its oxides in the colon have been made in health and ulcerative colitis. Nitrogen gas production in the colon of ulcerative colitis is significantly higher than in control cases[40] an observation that suggests greater denitrification in ulcerative colitis. The work was reported in 1949 but not re-examined since then. Further concern with the study is that N_2 was not directly measured and some cases of colitis may not have been of the ulcerative colitis type. The levels of nitrite (NO_2) in the rectum were first measured by placing saline-filled dialysis bags in the rectum by proctoscope after the rectum was reduced of bacteria.[41] Healthy subjects and acute and quiescent colitis cases were recruited. The level of nitrite was high in active colitis but not quiescent colitis. This observation was confirmed either by measuring gaseous nitric

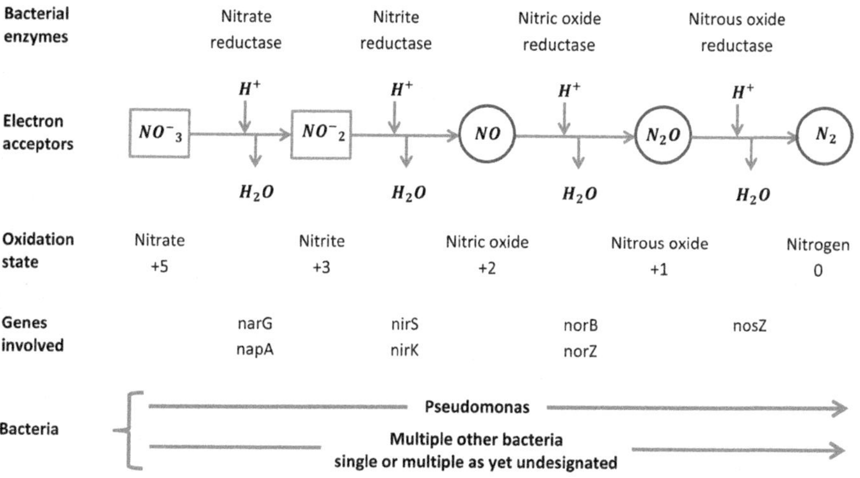

Figure 7.2 Features of anaerobic bacterial denitrification. □ = soluble salts, ○ = gaseous products. Numerous undesignated bacteria are involved in these processes.

oxide at colonoscopy(42, 43) or in serum or urine of cases of inflammatory bowel disease in children.(44) Direct needle probe investigation have also confirmed excess nitric oxide production in the mucosa of ulcerative colitis.(45) All the above methods ensured minimal presence of bacteria and therefore excluded nitric oxide contribution by bacteria of the colon. In the above experiments no excess nitric oxide production was found in quiescent colitis.

Measuring nitric oxide in the rectum that was not cleared of bacteria was undertaken by placing a balloon catheter in the rectum.(46, 47) This study confirmed elevated production of nitric oxide in active colitis but found in addition excessive production of nitric oxide in quiescent colitis. An explanation for this is that excessive production of nitric oxide in quiescent colitis would have originated from bacterial production of nitric oxide. Subsequently it has been confirmed that anaerobic colonic bacteria grown in culture produce nitric oxide when exposed to sodium nitrite.(48, 49)

The above observations permit a diagrammatic presentation (Fig. 7.3) showing that aerobic nitric oxide originates from the mucosa and

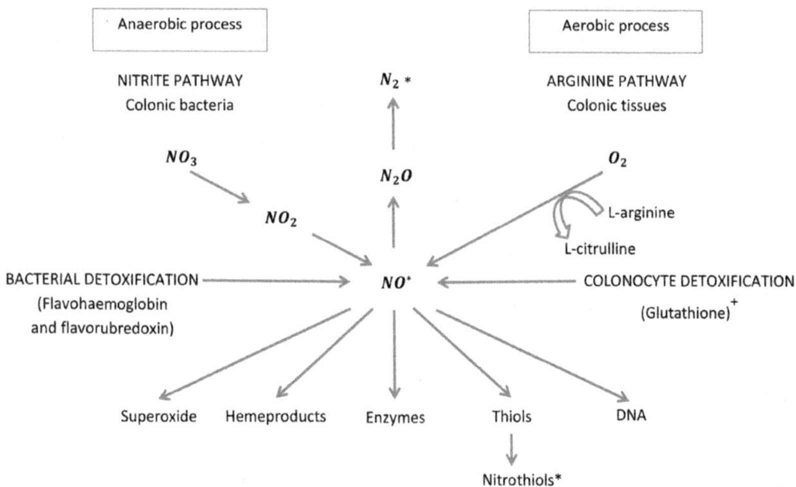

Figure 7.3 The bacterial 'anaerobic pathway' and tissue 'aerobic pathway' in the production of nitric oxide.
* products increased in ulcerative colitis, and
\+ = product reduced in ulcerative colitis.

anaerobic production of nitric oxide originates from bacteria via the process of denitrification as outlined earlier.

Having analysed the place of nitrogen in the human colon together with measurements of nitric oxide in ulcerative colitis it became possible to analyse whether nitrogenous agents particular ammonia, nitrite or nitric oxide played a role in the development of the biochemical lesions of ulcerative colitis.

AMMONIA: The predominant assimilatory derivative of bacterial nitrogen is ammonia (NH_3). Proposals have been made that ammonia is injurious to animal cells(50) or not injurious(51) yet colonic levels of ammonia are not elevated in mild or moderate ulcerative colitis.(52) Ammonia does not significantly alter cell respiration or metabolism of healthy human colonocytes.(53)

NITRITE/NITRIC OXIDE: Functionally nitrite enhances sodium absorption particularly in the distal colon.(54) These observations are however from animal work. With human colonocytes sodium nitrite strongly enhances butyrate oxidation to CO_2 but at the same time diminishes ketogenesis from butyrate.(55) Adding up all the oxidative products from butyrate oxidation in colonocytes exposed to nitrite, the total sum of oxidative products was diminished. This was a paradoxical observation that indicated that nitrite was subtly deleterious to colonocytes. Continuous exposure of the colon(55) to nitrite produced a 'no response' state referred to as a tachyphylaxis.

Thus nitrogenous products appear to play a central function in colonic bacterial metabolism and colonic sodium absorption. In addition nitrite causes subtle impairment of colonocyte metabolism.

7. The combined action of nitric oxide and sulphide on colonocytes

As neither sulphide alone nor nitric oxide alone could reproduce the biochemical lesions of ulcerative colitis in human colonocytes, experiments with these agents together were conducted. The reason for this combination was based on several biochemical and clinical clues suggesting that a combined action might be more profound in producing a biochemical change leading to biochemical lesions in colonocytes.

(i) Sulphide groups, predominantly those of cysteine, promote the effectiveness of nitric oxide in inducing relaxation of muscle(56, 57) probably through nitrosothiol formation. In the absence of sulphide groups nitric oxide is ineffective in promoting muscle relaxation. Sulphide groups thus promote the functional activity of nitric oxide in biological systems. The combined effect of nitric oxide and sulphide on butyrate oxidation was therefore tested in human colonocytes.

(ii) Sulphides are known to inhibit the final steps of bacterial denitrification (Fig. 7.4) at least in anaerobically grown cultures of *Pseudomonas*(58) or in bacterial sludges.(59) It was conceivable that sulphide might promote the accumulation of nitric oxide in a bacterial fermentative system such as the colon. The sulphide effect on nitric oxide production by human colonic bacteria has been tested in culture systems(60) which confirmed that cysteine and sulphides increase bacterial nitric oxide production more than forty-fold (Fig. 7.4). Under these conditions very high nitric oxide levels are

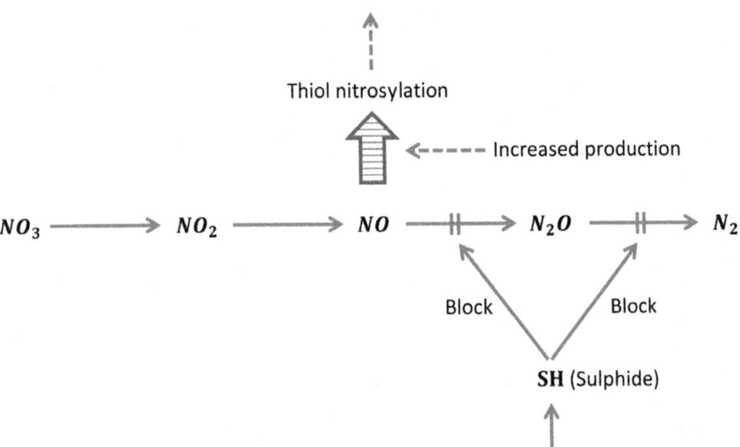

Figure 7.4 Action of 'sulphide' on the denitrification pathway. Sulphide gives enhanced nitric oxide production in fermentative systems and the colon.

achievable in the colon and may exceed the capacity of colonocytes to detoxify all the nitric oxide (Chapter 6).

Further experiments were therefore conducted with normal human colonocytes in the presence of sulphide and nitric oxide which was obtained from the nitric oxide donor S-nitrosoglutathione.[(61)] A combination of sulphide/nitric oxide reduced butyrate oxidation, ketogenesis and lowed acetyl CoA levels precisely as observed in the biochemical lesions of ulcerative colitis. Whether or not nitric oxide limited or inhibited lipid synthesis for cell membrane assembly was not known. To test this possibility an alternative cell system of isolated liver cells, referred to as hepatocytes,[(62)] were used and exposed to a nitric oxide donor. Added nitric oxide profoundly inhibited fatty acid and cholesterol synthesis in hepatocytes.[(62)] It is possible that such a response in colonocytes, not as yet tested, would produce cell membrane changes like that observed in electron micrographs of ulcerative colitis.[(63)]

Conclusions

The long and circuitous route of trying to imitate the 'biochemical lesions' of colonocytes in ulcerative colitis has led to the conclusion that bacteria and their metabolic products are central to the causation of ulcerative colitis. From the observations in this chapter three factors are a key to the onset of the biochemical lesions of colonocytes in ulcerative colitis.

(i) A specific complement of anaerobic denitrifying bacteria of which *E. coli*, *Pseudomonas*[58] and sulphate-reducing bacteria are examples. Sulphate reducing bacteria, despite their name are able to denitrify[64, 65, 66] and add to overall bacterial production of nitric oxide. Precise studies of denitrifying bacteria in the human colon still need to be undertaken probably with the help of environmental microbiologists.

(ii) A high content of nitrogen in food components (Chapter 8) of the diet is needed to provide the substrates for denitrification and the excess production of nitric oxide.

(iii) A high intake of sulphur containing amino acids is needed to provide the substrates for sulphide production by bacteria in the colon (Chapter 8).

The summative effect of the above three factors produces 'nitrosative stress' in the colon, that is excessive nitric oxide acting on colonocytes, for which the colonocyte capacity of detoxification by glutathione is not adequate. In contrast the detoxification capacity for NO by bacteria is enormous due to specific and unique mechanisms[67, 68] which provide tolerance of high concentrations of NO and thereby continuing bacterial growth.

An explanatory note on the evaluations of colonic bacteria in ulcerative colitis in light of the above findings is now appropriate. Studies of colonic bacteria over the last 120 years has been problematic. The methods of biochemical identification[69] and culture identification have led to new endeavours of genetic identification[70, 71] which in recent years has been marked by many reports published in the high profile journals *Nature* and *Science*. All three methods of identification however have a failing in that they do not accurately define the output of metabolites by bacteria and do not address the vital factor of 'quorum sensing' which is the self regulation of bacteria and bacterial growth as found in the colon.

Despite these weaknesses, a perceived limitation of analysis may provide the stimulus for future research and possibly unexpected findings in a complex bacterial system. The colonic bacterial system is now termed a 'microbiome', a gentler term than the historical description of colonic bacteria. Studies on the microbiome have progressed[72] but to date no central theme regarding the genetics of bacteria or bacterial metabolite production in ulcerative colitis has emerged.

References

1. Breuer RI, Buto SK, Christ ML et al. Rectal irrigation with short-chain fatty acids for distal ulcerative colitis. Dig Dis Sci. 36:185–7 (1991)
2. Scheppach W, Sommer H, Kirchner T et al. Effect of butyrate enemas on the colonic mucosa in distal ulcerative colitis. Gastroenterology 103:51- 6 (1992)
3. Hamer HM, Jonkers D, Venema K et al. Review article: the role of butyrate on colonic function. Aliment Pharmacol Therap 27:104–119 (2008)
4. Roediger WEW, Heyworth M, Willoughby P et al. Luminal ions and short chain fatty acids as markers of functional activity of the mucosa in ulcerative colitis. J. Clin. Path 35:323–326 (1982)
5. Treem WR, Ahsan N, Shoup M et al. Fecal short chain fatty acids in children with inflammatory bowel disease. J. Pediatr. Gastroenterol Nutr 18:159–164 (1994)
6. Thibault R, De Coppet P, Daly K et al. Down-regulation of the monocarboxylate transporter 1 is involved in butyrate deficiency during intestinal inflammation. Gastroenterology 133:1916–27 (2007)
7. Thibault R, Blachier F, Darcy-Vrillon B et al. Butyrate utilization by the colonic mucosa in inflammatory bowel diseases: a transport deficiency. Inflamm. Bowel Dis 16:684–695 (2010)
8. Roediger WEW. The place of short-chain fatty acids in colonocyte metabolism in health and ulcerative colitis: the impaired colonocyte barrier pp. 337–351 in Physiological and Clinical Aspects of Short-chain Fatty Acids. Eds JH Cummings, JL Rombeau and T Sakata. Cambridge University Press (1995)
9. Allan ES, Winter S, Light AM et al. Mucosal enzyme activity for butyrate oxidation; no defect in patients with ulcerative colitis. GUT 38:886–893 (1996)
10. Santhanam S, Venkatraman A, Ramakrishna BS. Impairment of mitochondrial acetoacetyl CoA thiolase activity in the colonic mucosa of patients with ulcerative colitis. GUT 56:1543–9 (2007)
11. DePreter V, Arijs I, Windey K et al. Impaired butyrate oxidation in ulcerative colitis is due to decreased butyrate uptake and a defect in the oxidation pathway. Inflam. Bowel Dis. 18:1127–36 (2012)
12. Sabbagh ED, Cuebas D and Schulz H. 3-Mercaptopropionic acid, a potent inhibitor of fatty acid oxidation in rat heart mitochrondia. J.Biol.Chem. 260:7337–7342 (1985)
13. Roediger WEW and Nance S. Selective reduction of fatty acid oxidation in colonocytes: correlation with ulcerative colitis. LIPIDS 25:642–652 (1990)
14. Duncan A, Kapaniris O, Roediger WEW. Measurement of mercaptoacetate levels in anaerobic batch culture of colonic bacteria. FEMS Microbiol. Ecol. 74:303–308 (1990)

15. Roediger WEW and Nance S. Metabolic induction of experimental ulcerative colitis by inhibition of fatty acid oxidation. Br J.Exp. Path. 67:773–782 (1986)
16. Cummings JH, Rombeau JL and Sakata, T. Physiological and clinical aspects of short-chain fatty acids. Cambridge University Press, Cambridge (1995)
17. Gibson GR, Cummings JH and Macfarlane GT et al. Alternative pathways for hydrogen disposal during fermentation in the human colon. GUT 31:679–83 (1990)
18. Pitcher MCL, Beatty ER and Cummings JH .The contribution of sulphate reducing bacteria and 5-aminosalicylic acid to faecal sulphide in patients with ulcerative colitis. GUT 46:64–72 (2000)
19. Gibson GR, Cummings JH and Macfarlane GT. Growth and activities of sulphate-reducing bacteria in gut contents from healthy subjects and patients with ulcerative colitis. FEMS Microbiol. Ecol. 9:103–112 (1991)
20. Rowan F, Docherty NG, Murphy M et al. Desulfvibrio bacterial species are increased in ulcerative colitis. Dis Colon Rectum 53:1530–1536 (2010)
21. Moore J, Babidge W and Roediger WEW. Colonic luminal hydrogen sulphide is not elevated in ulcerative colitis. Dig Dis Sciences 43:162–165 (1998)
22. Roediger WEW, Duncan A, Kapaniris O et al. Reducing sulphur compounds of the colon impair colonocyte nutrition: implications for ulcerative colitis. Gastroenterology 104:802–809 (1993)
23. Magee EA, Richardson CJ, Hughes R et al. Contribution of dietary protein to sulfide production in the large intestine: an in vitro and a controlled feeding study in humans. Am.J. Clin. Nutr. 72:1488–94 (2000)
24. Jowett SL, Seal CJ, Pearce MS et al. Influence of dietary factors on the clinical course of ulcerative colitis: a prospective cohort study. GUT 53:1479:1484 (2004)
25. Roediger WEW, Duncan A. 5-aminosalicylic acid decreases colonic sulphide formation: implications for ulcerative colitis. Med.Sci.Res. 24:27–29 (1996)
26. Moore JWE, Babidge WJ, Roediger WEW. Thiolmethyltransferase activity in the human colonic mucosa: implications for ulcerative colitis. J.Gastroeneterol.Hepat. 12:678–684 (1997)
27. Picton R, Eggo MC, Merrill GA et al. Mucosal protection against sulphide: importance of the enzyme rhodanese. GUT 50:201–205 (2002)
28. Ramasamy S, Singh S, Taniere P. Sulfide-detoxifying enzymes in the human colon are decreased in cancer and upregulated in differentiation. Am.J.Physiol. 291:G288-G286 (2006)
29. Thomas GAO, Rhodes J, Green JT et al. Role of smoking in inflammatory bowel disease: implications for therapy. Postgrad Med J 76:273–279 (2000)
30. Linden DR. Hydrogen sulfide signaling in the gastrointestinal tract. Antioxidants and Redox Signaling 20:818–830 (2014)
31. Keeney DR and Hatfield J. The nitrogen cycle, historical perspective and current and potential future concerns pp. 1–18 in 'Nitrogen in the environment. Sources, Problems and Management'. 2nd Edition Eds. Hatfield J + Follett RF. Academic Press/Elsevier, London (2008)
32. Wallace GI and Neave SL. The nitrite test as applied to bacterial cultures. J.Bacteriol. 14:377–384 (1927)
33. McFaddin J. Nitrate reduction test pp. 236–245 in Biochemical tests for identification of medical bacteria. 2nd Edition J. McFaddin. Williams and Wilkins, Baltimore (1980)
34. Payne WJ. Denitrification. Wiley-Interscience, New York, (1981)

35. Roediger WEW and Radcliffe BC. Role of nitrite and nitrate as a redox couple in the rat colon. Gastroeneterology 94:915–922 (1988)
36. Radcliffe B, Deakin EJ, Roediger WEW. Effect of luminal or circulating nitrite on colonic ion movement. Am.J.Physiol. 253: G246-G252 (1987)
37. Witter JP and Balish E. Distribution and metabolism of ingested NO_{3-} and NO_{2-} in germfree and conventional-flora rats. App Environ Microbiol 38:861–869 (1979)
38. Witter JP, Gatley SJ, Balish E. Distribution of nitrogen-13 from labeled nitrate ($^{13}NO_3^-$) in humans and rats. Science 204:411–413 (1979)
39. Radcliffe BC, Hall C, Roediger WEW. Nitrite and nitrate levels in ileostomy effluent: effect of dietary change. Br. J Nutr. 61:323–330 (1989)
40. Kirk E. The quantity and composition of human flatus. Gastroenterology 12:782–794 (1949)
41. Roediger WEW, Lawson MJ, Nance SH et al. Detectable colonic nitrite levels in inflammatory bowel disease – mucosal or bacterial malfunction. Digestion 35:199–204 (1986)
42. Lundberg JO, Hellstrom PM, Lundberg JM et al. Greatly increased luminal nitric oxide in ulcerative colitis. Lancet 344:1673–4 (1994)
43. Rachmilewitz D, Eliakim R, Ackerman Z et al. Direct determination of colonic nitric oxide level – a sensitive marker of disease activity in ulcerative colitis. Am.J. Gastroenterol. 93:409–412 (1998)
44. Levine JJ, Pettei MJ, Valderrama E et al. Nitric oxide and inflammatory bowel disease: evidence for local intestinal production in children with active colonic disease. J.Pediat.Gastroenterol 26:34–38 (1998)
45. Iwashita E. Greatly increased mucosal nitric oxide in ulcerative colitis determined in situ by a novel nitric oxide selective micro-electrode. J.Gastroenterol. Hepatol 13:391–395 (1998)
46. Reinders CI, Herulf M, Ljung T et al. Rectal mucosal nitric oxide in differentiation of inflammatory bowel disease and irritable bowel syndrome. Clin.Gastrenterol. Hepatol 3:777 -783 (2005)
47. Reinders CL, Jonkers D, Jansson EA et al. Rectal nitric oxide and fecal calprotectin in inflammatory bowel disease. Scand.J.Gastroeneterol 42:1151–1157 (2007)
48. Sobko T, Reinders CI, Jansson EA et al. Gastrointestinal bacteria generate nitric oxide from nitrate and nitrite. Nitric Oxide Biol Chem 13:272–278 (2005)
49. Cutruzzola F. Bacterial nitric oxide synthesis. Biochim Biophys Acta 114:231–249 (1999)
50. Visek WJ. Some aspects of ammonia toxicity in animal cells. J.Dairy Sci 51:286–295 (1968)
51. Wrong OM. Nitrogen metabolism in the large intestine in mammalian nutrition and homeostasis. Pp 133–155, Eds. Wrong OM, Edmonds CJ, Chadwick VS, MTP Press, Lancaster (1981)
52. Roediger WEW, Heyworth M and Willoughby P et al. Luminal ions and short chain fatty acids as markers of functional activity of the mucosa in ulcerative colitis. J.Clin Path 35:323–326 (1982)
53. Roediger WEW. Role of anaerobic bacteria in the metabolic welfare of the colonic mucosa. GUT 21:793–798 (1980)
54. Roediger WEW, Deakin EJ, Radcliffe BC et al. Anion control of sodium absorption in the colon. Quart J Exp Physiol. 71:195–204 (1986)

55. Roediger WEW, Radcliffe BC, Deakin EJ et al. Specific metabolic effect of sodium nitrIte on fat metabolism by mucosal cells of the colon. Dig Dis Sci 31:535–539 (1986)
56. Ignarro LJ, Lippton H, Edwards JC et al. Mechanism of vascular smooth muscle relaxation by organic nitrates, nitrites, nitroprusside and nitric oxide. Evidence for the involvement of S-nitrosothiols as active intermediates. J.Pharmacol.Exp Ther 218:739–749 (1981)
57. Hosoki R, Matsuki N and Kimura H. The possible role of hydrogen sulphide as an endogenous smooth muscle relaxant in synergy with nitric oxide. Biochem Biophys Res Com. 237:527–531 (1997)
58. Sorenson J, Tiedje JM and Firestone RB. Inhibition by sulphide of nitric and nitrous oxide reduction by denitrifying Pseudomonas fluorescens. Appl Environ Mircobiol 39:105–108 (1980)
59. Manconi I, van der Maas P and Lens PNL. Effect of sulfur compounds on biological reduction of nitric oxide in aqueous Fe(II) EDTA2- solutions. Nitric Oxide 15:40–49 (2006)
60. Vermeiren J, van de Wiele T, van Nieuwenhuyse G et al. Sulfide-and nitrite-dependent nitric oxide production in the intestinal tract. Microbiol Biotech 5:379–387 (2012)
61. Roediger WE, Babidge WJ. Nitric oxide effect on colonocyte metabolism: co-action of sulfides and peroxide. Mol Cell Biochem 206:159–167 (2000)
62. Roediger W, Hems R, Wiggins D et al. Inhibition of hepatocyte lipogenesis by nitric oxide donor: could nitric oxide regulate lipid synthesis. IUBMB Life 56:35–40 (2004)
63. Delpre G, Avidor I, Steinherz R et al. Ultrastructural abnormalities in endoscopically and histologically normal and involved colon in ulcerative colitis. Am J Gastroenterology 84:1038–1046 (1989)
64. Riederer-Henderson MA, Wilson PW. Nitrogen fixation by sulphate-reducing bacteria. J.Gen Microbiol 61:27–31 (1970)
65. Moura I, Bursakov S, Costa C et al. Nitrate and nitrite utilization in sulfate-reducing bacteria. Anaerobe 3:279–290 (1997)
66. Silaghi-Dumitrescu R, Yong K, Viswanathan R et al. A flavo-diiron protein from desulfovibrio vulgaris with oxidase and nitric oxide reductase activities. Evidence for an in vivo nitric oxide scavenging function. Biochem 44:3572–3579 (2005)
67. Poole RK. Nitric oxide and nitrosative stress tolerance in bacteria. Biochem Soc Trans 33:176–180 (2005)
68. Stern AM and Zhu J. An introduction to nitric oxide sensing and response in bacteria. Adv App Microbiol 87:187–220 (2014)
69. Macfaddin JF. Biochemical tests for identification of medical bacteria. Williams + Wilkins, Baltimore (1980)
70. The Human Microbiome Project Consortium. Structure function and diversity of the healthy human microbiome. Nature 486:207–214 (2012)
71. Balter M. Taking stock of the human microbiome and disease. Science 336:1246–1247 (2012)
72. Huttenhower C, Kostic AD and Xavier RJ. Inflammatory bowel disease as a model for translating the microbiome. Immunity 40:843–854 (2014)

-8-

Vascular and dietary sources of colonic nitrogen and sulphur

OUTLINE: Nitrogen in the circulation is extracted into the colon particularly when nitric oxide is elevated in infection elsewhere in the body. Crop fertilization hugely increases the nitrogen content of food, a process intensified after 1918 and after which ulcerative colitis became more common. Nitrogen fertilization is very modest in Africa where ulcerative colitis is rare. The chief sulphide source is meat protein, high intake of which may precipitate an attack of ulcerative colitis.

Because the biochemical lesions in colonocytes could be mimicked by nitric oxide with sulphide it seemed worthwhile to further consider the nitrogen and sulphur input into the colon.

Nitrogen sources

Nitrogen input into the colon from the luminal aspect has in part been detailed in the previous chapter. More pertinent now is the phenomenon of transmucosal entry of nitrate when administered intravenously.[1] Any elevation of circulating nitrate/nitrite given intravenously not only elevates urinary excretion of these but much nitrite is found in the lumen of the caecum and colon. These findings are of relevance to ulcerative colitis particularly where conditions such as infection beyond the colon, for example, pneumonia may raise the circulating nitric oxide/nitrate levels which would be taken up in the colon.[2] Such nitrogen uptake is associated with exacerbation of active ulcerative colitis[3] an observation long known but not clearly explained.

With regard to luminal nitrogen level the main factor is the degree of nitration observed in foods, particularly vegetables. This is dependent on the method of growth, the hours of sunlight and the use of nitrogen fertilizer. It was von Liebig who in 1840 analysed the composition of vegetation[4] and found mainly carbon, nitrogen and mineral salts. There appeared no insufficiency in carbon while the nitrogen content was very variable being either high or low in levels. While atmospheric N_2 is plentiful it is not in an assimilable form for plants. Liebig developed a means of applying nitrogen to plants at the roots via ammonia salts. Soil bacteria convert ammonia salt to nitrate and nitrite. Nitrogen application doubles and quadruples crop yields. Between 1840 and 1920 guano and nitrate salts were used as a form of nitrogen application[5] but after 1918 the Haber-Bosch process[6] which converted nitrogen gas to usable nitrogen (ammonium chloride) took over from nitrate salts. The utilization of nitrogen fertilizer increased from 340,000 tons to 86 million tons between 1901 and 2001. While the world population increased from 1.65 billion to 6.06 billion over the same time period.[5] The Haber-Bosch derived nitrogen was abundantly used in Europe, UK and USA while hardly at all in Africa.[7] The international Fertilizer Industry Association (IFA) in 2014 indicated that in Africa less than 10 kg per hectare fertilizer is used in contrast with more than a global value of 100 kg/hectare in the developed countries. The cropped plants in rural Africa are known to be nitrogen poor.[7] The phenomenon of nitrogen fertilization parallels the high incidence of ulcerative colitis in UK/Europe/USA, compared with Africa where there is a very low incidence of ulcerative colitis.[8,9] The IOIBD (International Organisation of Inflammatory Bowel Disease) survey of ulcerative colitis parallels the rate of nitrogen fertilization throughout the world.[9] The correlation of disease prevalence of ulcerative colitis and rates of nitrogen fertilization are not proven but many leads converge to make this a plausible explanation.

Sulphur sources

The biology of sulphide metabolism in the colon has been detailed earlier (Chapter 7). In dietary terms the amount of meat protein ingested will raise the colonic sulphide levels.[10] Other foods that may do this too are eggs, cheese, milk and vegetables with a high sulphur amino acid content particularly cruciferous vegetables. Much further work needs to be done in this regard but diets[11] and medication such as 5-amino salicylic acid that reduce the sulphide content in the colon lead to considerable improvement of ulcerative colitis. It has also been noted that diets high in sulphur amino acids are the cause of relapse of ulcerative colitis.[12] In the book

Fear of Food[13] many dietary factors of concern have been enumerated but the concept of excess nitrogen and sulphide in the colon has not been previously considered. The therapeutic implications of nitrogen and sulphide in the colon will be discussed in the next chapter.

References

1. Witter JP, Gatley SJ and Balish E. Distribution of nitrogen-13 labeled nitrate ($^{13}NO_3$-) in humans and rats. Science 204:401–413 (1979)
2. Roediger WEW. Nitric oxide damage to colonocytes in colitis-by-association: remote transfer of nitric oxide to the colon. Digestion: 65:191–195 (2002)
3. Mee AS, Jewell DP. Factors inducing relapse in inflammatory bowel disease. Br Med J ii:801–802 (1978)
4. Liebig BJ. Chemistry and its application to Agriculture and Physiology. 4th Edition, pp. 3–4. Eds. Playfair L. and Gregory W. Taylor and Walton, London (1847)
5. Cushman GT. Guano and the Opening of the Pacific World. Cambridge University Press, Cambridge (2013)
6. Smil V. Enriching the earth, Fritz Haber, Carl Bosch and the transformation of world food production. The MIT Press, Cambridge, Massachusetts (2001)
7. Charles D. Our fertilized world. National Geographic 223:94–110 (2013)
8. Kelly P and Sinkala E. The Gut pp. 656–670 in Principles of Medicine in Africa, 4th Edition. Eds Mabey D et al. Cambridge University Press, Cambridge UK (2013)
9. Ng SC, Bernstein CN, Vatn MH et al. Geographical variability and environmental risk factors in inflammatory bowel disease. GUT 62:630–649 (2013)
10. Magee EA, Richardson GJ, Hughes R et al. Contribution of dietary protein to sulfide production in the large intestine: an in vitro and a controlled feeding study in humans. Am J Clin Nutr 72:1488–94 (2000)
11. Roediger WEW. Decreased sulphur amino acid intake in ulcerative colitis. Lancet 351:1555 (1998)
12. Jowett SL, Seal CJ, Pearce MS et al. Influence of dietary factors on the clinical course of ulcerative colitis: a prospective cohort study. Gut 53:1479–1484 (2004)
13. Levenstein H. Fear of food. A history of why we worry about what we eat. University of Chicago Press, Chicago (2013)

-9-

Slow toxicity and colonic extent of ulcerative colitis

OUTLINE: Toxins are classed as fast or slow. NO+SH acts as a slow toxin and regional manifestation of disease depends on exposure time. Progression of ulcerative colitis in the colon is related to these factors.

One of the most perplexing manifestations of ulcerative colitis is the siting of the initial disease, usually the rectum, and subsequent progression along the colon as well as the observation of skip lesions in the colon.[1] If nitric oxide in conjunction with sulphide are causative of ulcerative colitis, as yet only partially verified, then how in terms of toxicology do these agents impact on colonocytes in the colon?

To answer this question we need to solicit the help of toxicological conventions. The division of toxins is often made into 'fast' or 'slow' toxins.[2] Fast toxins are observed by escalating the dose until a toxic biochemical feature is demonstrated. A prime example of this is the use of escalating doses of sodium sulphide acting on isolated human colonocytes.[3] This method is often used to find the 'lethal' dose of an agent. Damage with sulphide was observed in healthy human colonocytes but the damage was not comparable with the biochemical lesions observed in human ulcerative colitis.

The invocation of 'slow toxins' has much greater relevance to ulcerative colitis than 'fast' toxins. Slow toxins can cause changes in several different ways. Toxins can accumulate in colonocytes until cell levels become sufficiently high to cause cell injury or there may be a process of non accumulation where the progressive increment of damage either as genetic damage or by progressive sequestration of, for instance, CoA may cause metabolic changes in colonocytes. Toxicologists verify damaging results by undertaking subchronic or chronic tests in experimental animals. Tests invoke finer points such as the route of administration, the animal species used and the number of animals used. More important is the dose selection and the duration of experiments. The convention for chronic toxicity is the 90 days study in small animals. Such a chronic study employing nitric oxide and sulphide has not yet been done in animals and would, because of the very high costs of nitric oxide donors, be extremely difficult to undertake. The route of administration would probably be best by direct colonic instillation as has previously been done for nitrite instillation in the animal colon.(4)

With regard to the colon several of the above toxicological principles have application. The dose of nitric oxide may vary with dietary manipulation and the nature of the bacterial enterotype in the colon.(5) The sulphide level likewise, is dependent on dietary factors and prevailing enterotype.(6) The important factor is the duration of contact of microbial metabolites with the colonic mucosa. This would depend on the time of colonic transit of luminal contents. Many cases of ulcerative colitis have an antecendent history of constipation either distal colonic hold up or generalized slow transit through the colon. Constipation may cause prolonged mucosal exposure to microbial metabolites. The distal colon is most prone to prolonged exposure to microbial metabolites and is where ulcerative colitis manifests most frequently. Another site of bacterial stasis may be the appendiceal lumen which leads to peri-appendiceal inflammation in a proportion of cases of ulcerative colitis.(7) The peri-appendiceal inflammation has mostly been observed at colonoscopy, a finding that has emerged in the last 30 years. Peri-appendiceal orifice inflammation has been described as a 'skip' lesion in ulcerative colitis and has lead to the proposal that appendicectomy may be therapeutic in the treatment of ulcerative colitis.(8) This proposal has remained controversial.

The progression of colitis more proximal from the initiating site of rectum or rectosigmoid can be explained metabolically on the basis of (1) progressive sequestration of CoA and (2) an impaired capacity to detoxify nitric oxide. Impaired detoxification of phenol(9) and sulphide(10) by colonocytes in ulcerative colitis has already been mentioned previously. The capacity of colonocytes to detoxify nitric oxide via glutathione is very limited and peak capacity to detoxify nitric oxide would be rapidly reached in the presence of chronic high levels of nitric oxide.

In conclusion the siting of the disease of ulcerative colitis, in addition to the previously described denitrifying bacteria, in the setting of a high nitrogen intake and a high sulphur intake, also requires the action of 'slow toxins' at the sites where there is a prolonged contact with the damaging metabolites of nitric oxide and sulphide. Prolonged contact is mostly in the distal colon. Proximal progression of the disease would occur depending on the capacity of colonocytes to detoxify nitric oxide and sulphide. Therapeutic options to minimize the putative causative agents of ulcerative colitis, that is nitric oxide and sulphide, are detailed in the next chapter.

References

1. Joo M and Odze D. Rectal sparing and skip lesions in ulcerative colitis: a comparative study of endoscopic and histologic findings in patients who underwent proctocolectomy. Am J Surg Pathol. 34:689–696 (2010)
2. Rodricks JV. Calculated risks. The toxicity and human health risks of chemicals in our environment. Cambridge University Press, (1994)
3. Roediger WEW, Duncan A, Kapaniris O et al. Reducing sulfur compounds of the colon impair colonocyte nutrition: implications for ulcerative colitis. Gastroenterology 104:802–809 (1993)
4. Roediger WEW, Radcliffe BC, Deakin EJ et al. Specific metabolic effect of sodium nitrite on fat metabolism by mucosal cells of the colon. Dig Dis Sci 31:535–539 (1986)
5. Wu GD, Hoffmann C, Billinger K et al. Linking long-term dietary patterns with gut microbial enterotypes. Science 334:105–108 (2011)
6. Magee EA, Richardson GJ, Hughes R et al. Contribution of dietary protein to sulphide production in the large intestine: an in vitro and a controlled feeding study in humans. Am J Clin.Nutri. 72:1488–94 (2000)
7. Park SH, Loftus EV and Yang SK. Appendiceal skip inflammation and ulcerative colitis. Dig Dis Sci 59:2050–2057 (2014)
8. Bolin T, Wong S, Crouch R et al. Appendicectomy as a therapy for ulcerative proctitis. Am J Gastroenterol 104:2476–2482 (2009)
9. Ramakrishna BS, Roberts-Thomson IC and Roediger WEW. Impaired sulphation of phenol by the colonic mucosa in quiescent and active colitis. Gut 32:46–49 (1991)
10. De Preter V, Arijs I, Windey K et al. Decreased mucosal sulfide detoxification is related to an impaired butyrate oxidation in ulcerative colitis. Inflamm Bowel Dis 18:2371–2380 (2012)

-10-

Treatment of the precipitating factors of ulcerative colitis. The concept of bioremediation

OUTLINE: Dietary change and 5-aminosalicyclic acid reduce colonic sulphide formation. Immune suppression reduces nitric oxide production from activated immune cells. Oral antibiotics, single or multiple, provide improvement of ulcerative colitis presumably by decreasing bacterial nitric oxide production. Bioremediation by various means holds promise for future treatment of ulcerative colitis.

If the causation of ulcerative colitis can accurately be predicted then therapeutic benefits by targeting the newly perceived disease processes should ensue. Treatment of ulcerative colitis in the past was based on empirical principles using salazopyrin or countering inflammation with prednisolone. Treatment of the inflammatory response together with treatment of the causative factors should provide better outcomes in the management of ulcerative colitis than previously by empirical means only. Treatment to reduce the bacterial production of sulphide and nitric oxide are highlighted below.

Diminishing sulphide production

1. 5-ASA

5-aminosalicylic acid, the active component of salazopyrin[1] and one of the most frequently used and efficacious drugs for ulcerative colitis, reduces the fermentative production of sulphide from sulphur amino acids.[2] This observation, first reported in Adelaide in 1996, was rapidly confirmed by studies in the UK.[3,4] Diminishing sulphide levels reduces the amplification of nitric oxide production in the colonic lumen[5] and thereby diminishes epithelial cell damage. In the colon little of the salazopyrin is absorbed and 5-ASA is acetylated by colonocytes[6] to an inactive form of the drug. A continuous supply of 5-ASA is needed for ongoing suppression of sulphide formation in the colon.

2. *Diet*

Restricting the dietary intake of sulphur amino acids produces symptomatic improvement and reduction of stool frequency in established ulcerative colitis.[7] Direct measurements of sulphide reduction have not been made with this diet nevertheless high meat intake does raise the sulphide content of the colon.[8] Vegetables of the cruciferous variety may have a high content of sulphur amino acids and thereby raise the colonic content of sulphide, a point particularly applicable to vegetarians.

Diminishing nitric oxide production

1. *From activated immune cells*

The standard medications for ulcerative colitis such as prednisolone, azathioprine, methotrexate and a range of biologicals reduce the action of activated immune cells and thereby the reduction of nitric oxide as well as harmful cytokines produced by inflammatory cells. Current elucidations of the causation of ulcerative colitis recognizes inflammatory cell production of nitric oxide in the disease process (see Fig. 7.3) treatment of which was introduced after the mid 1950s starting with the use of prednisolone.[9]

Another agent reducing nitric oxide of activated immune cells is curcumin[10] which has been used in open treatment trials of ulcerative colitis[11] and found to maintain remission of ulcerative colitis. Placebo controlled trials have not yet been done.

2. *From bacterial denitrification*

Inhibiting the denitrifying enzyme activity of denitrification has been applied in agriculture to limit nitric oxide production from fertilizer and thereby limit the loss of N_2 gas into the atmosphere. Antibiotics are known to inhibit enzymes[12] in the denitrification pathway but similar applications have not yet been done in the human colon[13] of ulcerative colitis. The role of antibiotic effectiveness[14] in suppression of denitrification in the colon is currently under-explored, nevertheless lessons of past use of antibiotics in ulcerative colitis pose a hopeful prospect.

(i) Short term use of single antibiotics

Oral utilization of non-absorbable antibiotic such as tobramycin in the treatment of ulcerative colitis[15] was a bold therapeutic venture as use of antibiotics are prone to causing diarrhoea, complicating symptoms of ulcerative colitis. Burke and colleagues showed that tobramycin significantly assisted the remission of active ulcerative colitis[15] but did not have a lasting effect after 2 years.[16] Tobramycin is particularly active against *Pseudomonas* organisms that are powerful denitrifying bacteria. Presumably the short term use of tobramycin did not completely eradicate all denitrifying bacteria and hence failed to control ulcerative colits in the long term.

(ii) Use of multiple antibiotics – short term, long term

A multicentre study of triple antibiotics (ampicillin, tetracycline and metronidazole) for 2 weeks[17] was used in steroid dependent cases of ulcerative colitis. More than 60% of cases were able to stop steroids and follow up after 12 months showed maintenance of improvement unlike with the cases of single antibiotic use. A similar improvement with oral amoxicillin and doxycyline was reported in a group of paediatric patients with severe ulcerative colitis.[18]

(iii) Denitrification inhibitors

The concept to reduce nitrogen losses in soils brings the benefit of prolonged efficiency of fertilizer for the growth of plants and crops. The inhibition of converting ammonia to nitrate by the nitrification inhibitor nitrapyrin[19] has been achieved. This agent, in theory, would reduce the formation of nitrate for the denitrification pathway. Nitrapyrin is non toxic to humans but has not been tested in ulcerative colitis. The direct inhibition of denitrification[20] has only been tested in soils but may have application for ulcerative colitis.

Bioremediation – altering bacterial enterotypes

Originally 'bioremediation' was used as an umbrella term for an array of methods of waste water management. In a broader sense it implies replacing harmful bacteria by promoting growth or replacement of bacteria that are not harmful.[21] Certainly in ulcerative colitis denitrification and amplification of nitric oxide production by sulphide formation could be considered the result of 'harmful bacteria' but this has not been taken to animal models to verify. The harmful/harmless bacterial concept is notional yet has remained alive for more than a hundred years.[22] The concept has provided a drive to measure and modify bacteria in the colon. These include:

1. Microbiome studies, that is a genetic profile of the types and distribution of bacteria that might cause inflammation in the colon
2. Use of probiotics, that is ingestion of live bacteria[23] often lactobacilli
3. Use of prebiotics, that is ingestion of substrates for bacteria to proliferate in the colon
4. Use of symbiotics, that is a combination of pre and probiotics[24]
5. Use of human faecal transplants particularly in ulcerative colitis

Carefully randomized and controlled studies for all of the above are still being awaited. In the main the concept of harmful and harmless bacteria, as well as auto-intoxication, are as topical today (2016) as they were one hundred years ago.

References

1. Azad Khan AK, Piris J, Truelove SC. An experiment to determine the active therapeutic moiety of sulphasalazine. Lancet 310:892–5 (1977)
2. Roediger WEW and Duncan A. 5-ASA decreases colonic sulphide formation: implications for ulcerative colitis. Med Sci Res 24:27–9 (1996)
3. Pitcher MCL, Beatty ER and Cummings JH. The contribution of sulphate reducing bacteria and 5-aminosalicylic acid to faecal sulphide in patients with ulcerative colitis. Gut 46:64–72 (2000)
4. Edmond LM, Magee EA and Cummings JH. The effect of 5-aminosalicyclic acid containing drugs on sulphide production by sulphate-reducing and amino acid-fermenting bacteria. Inflam Bow Dis 9:10–17 (2003)
5. Vermeiren J, van de Wiele T, van Nieuwenhuyse G et al. Sulfide-and nitrite-dependent nitric oxide production in the intestinal tract. Microb Biotech 5:379–387 (2012)
6. Ireland A, Priddle JD, Jewell DP. Acetylation of 5-aminosalicyclic acid by isolated human colonic epithelial cells. Clin Sci 78:105–111 (1990)
7. Roediger WEW. Decreased sulphur amino acid intake in ulcerative colitis. Lancet 351:1555 (1998)
8. Magee EA, Hughes R and Cummings JH. Contribution of dietary protein to sulfide production in the large intestine: an invitro and a controlled feeding study in humans. Am J Clin Nutri 72:1488–1494 (2000)

9. Kirsner's Inflammatory Bowel Disease 6th Ed. Ed Sartor RB and Sandborn WJ. Saunders Edinburgh (2004)
10. Sreejay AN and Rao MNA. Nitric oxide scavenging by curcuminoids. J Pharm Pharmacol 49:105–107 (1997)
11. Vikas S, Pratap Mouli V, Garg SK et al. Induction with NCB-02 (Curcumin) enema for mild-to-moderate distal ulcerative colitis-a randomized placebo-controlled pilot study. J Crohns Colitis 8:208–214 (2014)
12. Murray RE and Knowles R. Chloramphenicol inhibition of denitrifying enzyme activity in two agricultural soils. App Env Microbiol 65:3487–3492 (1999)
13. Moir JWB. Bacterial nitrogen cycling in the human body pp. 233–247 in Nitrogen Cycling in Bacteria Molecular Analysis Ed JWB Moir. Caister Academic Press (2011)
14. Laximinarayan R. Antibiotic effectiveness: balancing conservation against innovation. Science 345:1299–1304 (2014)
15. Burke DA, Axon AT, Clayden SA et al. The efficacy of tobramycin in the treatment of ulcerative colitis. Aliment Pharmacol Ther 4:123–129 (1990)
16. Lobo AJ, Burke DA, Sobala GM et al. Oral tobramcyin in ulcerative colitis: effect on maintenance of remission. Alimen. Pharmacol Ther 7:155–158 (1993)
17. Kato K, Ohkusa T, Terao S et al. Adjunct antibiotic combination therapy for steroid-refactory or-dependent ulcerative colitis: an open-label multicentre study. Aliment Pharmacol Ther 39:949–956 (2014)
18. Turner D, Levine A, Kolho K-L et al. Combination of oral antibiotics may be effective in severe pediatric ulcerative colitis: a preliminary report. J. Crohn's Col. 8:1464–1470 (2014)
19. Gao S, Pan WL and Koenig PT. Wheat root growth responses to enhanced curcumin supply. Soil Sci Soc Am J 62:1736–1740 (1998)
20. Bremner JM, Yeomans JC. Effects of nitrification inhibitors on denitrification of nitrate in soil. Biol Fert Soils 2:173–179 (1986)
21. Bioremediation. Science and Applications. Eds Skipper HD and Turco RF. Soil Sciences Society of America. Madison Wisconsin USA (1995)
22. Autointoxication and its discontents pp. 27–42 in Fear of Food. A history of why we worry about what we eat. H. Levenstein. The University of Chicago Press, Chicago (2013)
23. Sanders ME, Guarner F, Guerrant R et al. An update on the use and investigation of probiotics in health and disease. Gut 62:787–796 (2013)
24. Furrie E, Macfarlane S, Kennedy A et al. Synbiotic therapy (Bifidobacterium longum/Synergy 1) initiates resolution of inflammation in patients with active ulcerative colitis: a randomised controlled pilot trial. Gut 54:242–249 (2005)

-11-

Conclusions on the causation of ulcerative colitis – the strength of evidence

OUTLINE: Denitrifying bacteria of which *Pseudomonas* are an example, together with excessive bacterial production of sulphide and nitric oxide, are central to the causation of ulcerative colitis. Ulcerative colitis is a disease of nitrosative stress. Reproducibility of much of the work has yielded reliable knowledge. Further research into ulcerative colitis remains to be done.

Analysts of science and of the associated philosophy of science tend to categorize knowledge as either reliable[1] or uncertain.[2] The pathway taken in the foregoing chapters is based on quantifiable observations from biochemical experimentation. They are markers of distance travelled in the process of science towards unlocking causation of ulcerative colitis and reflect a positive reduction of uncertainty in knowledge. Reproducibility of experimental observations is one guideline of reliable knowledge: this has been achieved by the amplification and experimental reproduction of results by other scientists quoted in the preceding chapters. What lies on the uncertainty side of the ledger is the sequence of events that take place in the causation of ulcerative colitis. Immunologists will nominate immune activity as being the first act of the disease process: geneticists will put certain gene loci on the chromosome at the centre for producing metabolic changes and microbiologists will opt for microbial 'dysbiosis' as the primary event in the disease process. All scientists would have difficulty in separating initiating factors from propagating factors which in the colon would be problematic to answer. Perhaps we need the optimism and mind set of brilliant physicists. Albert Einstein and David Hilbert separately proposed the theory of relativity. Hilbert maintained 'there is no such thing as an unsolvable problem'.

The observations on the cause of ulcerative colitis can be put together as follows:

1. The colon is a fermentative chamber that requires microbial growth, an input of carbon, nitrogen, sulphur as well as bound oxygen (to nitrogen or sulphur) for bacterial respiration. Many resulting products are either solutes such as short chain fatty acids (butyrate) or volatile gaseous products (CH_4, NO, N_2, CO_2 or H_2S). Bacterial metabolites sustain and promote the welfare of colonic epithelial cells, reflecting an enduring symbiosis between humans and microbes. One cannot function without the other. Cellular welfare and microbial welfare are kept in tight balance. Both colonic epithelial cells and microbes have a wide latitude of tolerance to metabolic change (for example by detoxification) within which is ensured the welfare of each other.

2. The precise control of growth of a single microbial species in the presence of a large number of varying microbes is currently unknown but one regulating factor is the abundance of nitrogen and sulphur entering the fermentative chambers. The amount of carbon input into the colon has so far not been associated with disease manifestation and, as Liebig showed in 1840 for plants, the limiting elements now for microbial growth are nitrogen and sulphur.

3. Microbial denitrification is one factor of nitrogen control in the fermentative chamber in which process sulphide may impede the gaseous production of N_2 and lead to accumulation of nitric oxide which is poorly tolerated by colonocytes. Their capacity to detoxify nitric oxide is limited and a long exposure to nitric oxide from bacteria produces a 'slow toxin' response in epithelial cells. Lipid synthesis in colonocytes is impaired by nitric oxide as well as mucus production which normally provide an effective epithelial barrier against bacteria. The epithelial barrier is broken down by excessive bacterial nitric oxide. The scene is set for further damage to be caused by nitric oxide from activated immune cells brought about by lowered epithelial barrier function. The former symbiotic relationship between bacteria and colonocytes becomes degraded and immune cell activity prominently activated.

4. Another pathway of nitrogen handling in the colon is through potential production of ammonia which is far less injurious than nitric oxide and not affected by the presence of sulphide. A key question is: does denitrification or ammonification dominate in the human colon? From results so far it

would seem that denitrification dominates in ulcerative colitis but not in health. Further studies are needed to bring resolution to this proposal.

5. The bacteria most frequently studied with regard to denitrification are *Pseudomonas* species which have the enzyme complement to reduce nitrate to nitrogen gas. One antibiotic with specific action against *Pseudomonas* (tobramycin) (Chapter 10) has been of great therapeutic value in treating active ulcerative colitis. The road ahead would be to conduct more experiments on denitrifying bacteria in health and disease together with the effects of antibiotics on denitrifying bacteria.

If the experimental work now presented could be brought to a mathematical quantity it would then be possible to undertake a 'likelihood' assessment as promoted by Sir Ronald Fisher.[3] Likelihood is often substituted by 'probability' but is not quite equatable. A positive test of likelihood of the current scientific proposals would be a boon to secure a platform for future research.

Finally 'ideal' knowledge is often designated 'truth'.[4] An experimental observation is regarded as truthful when it corresponds with the facts of clinical disease. For this reason experiments were conducted with humans or human material both in health and those with ulcerative colitis. Numerous separate expressions of truth have been put forward in the previous chapters. The strength of evidence falls into separate expressions of truth. Hopefully the work presented will be durable and a means to the scientific road ahead.

References

1. Ziman JM. Reliable knowledge: an exploration of the grounds for belief in science. Cambridge University Press, Cambridge (1978)
2. Dolby RGA. Uncertain knowledge, an image of science for a changing world. Cambridge University Press, Cambridge (1996)
3. Fisher RA. Statistical methods for research workers 14th Edition. Oliver and Bagot, Edinburgh (1970)
4. Blackburn S and Simmons K (eds). Truth. Oxford University Press, Oxford (1999)

PART THREE

Crohn's Disease

-12-

A profusion of ideas for Crohn's disease

OUTLINE: Factors in genes, the state of the immune system and the state of bowel contents have been nominated for the causation of Crohn's disease. Genetic analysis has not unravelled a causative process. The immune system in Crohn's disease is activated though the cause of activation unknown. Strong clues have emerged for a luminal factor in the bowel in the causation of Crohn's disease. In the lumen microbes appear to play a part in causation and antibiotics at times have produced positive therapeutic responses.

The unknown has drawn speculation on the causation of Crohn's disease for which an abundance of ideas, both vague and exotic, have been put forward. A fistful of hypotheses have resulted such as toothpaste exposure, antibiotic exposure and a 'hygiene hypothesis' together with many other suggestions. None have satisfactorily fitted the cause for gut inflammation of the Crohn's variety.

The mantra in modern science literature is that Crohn's disease results from 'a dysregulated mucosal immune response to environmental factors in genetically susceptible hosts'.[1,2,3,4] Many state of the art reviews begin from this repetitive proposal which invokes (1) genetic make-up, (2) the immune system and (3) the environment. These are worthy of further consideration.

Genetic factors

Up to 20% of Crohn's cases occur in families, a statistic that has emerged in the last 30 years. Such concentration of disease has called into question a genetic predisposition and produced many analyses which have excluded single gene disorders, either by gene deletion or gene transposition, for Crohn's disease. So far approximately 160 susceptibility gene loci have been identified[5] and the risk loci highlighted pathways of innate immunity, adaptive immune responses, barrier function, pathogen sensing and response to oxidative stress. These observations have led to the conclusion that Crohn's disease is a multifactorial disease. Many other diseases such as diabetes and heart disease have a similar familial clustering and have multiple but different susceptibility genes. So far in Crohn's disease genetic analysis has not been able to unravel metabolic characteristics or defence weaknesses leading towards a causative process.(6)

Experts of genetic research have advanced that predictive genetic tests for hereditary diseases or repairing mutational genes will lead to radical breakthroughs in clinical medicine. To date this has not occurred in Crohn's disease though the huge financial investment in gene technology may lead to success in the future.

Immune Factors

The lamina propria of the gut mucosa is a diffuse immune system along the gastrointestinal tract. Regulation and dysregulation of immune receptors, immune cell function and cytokine patterns are topics that have burgeoned in the literature of Crohn's disease.(7) The pharmaceutical industry has targeted the immune system, some brochures designating Crohn's disease as an 'auto-immune disease'. Evidence for such a disease pattern has not been very strong. Nevertheless suppression of active inflammation by pharmaceutical means has brought undoubted improvement of Crohn's disease but not necessarily complete remission or prevention of recurrence of Crohn's disease. To date the antigen that activates the immune system in Crohn's disease has not been found and therefore prompts a closer look at the luminal environment of bacteria to seek out a potential trigger or triggers.

Environmental Factors

An experiment that supported environmental factors in the causation of Crohn's disease was conducted in Belgium with Crohn's patients undergoing surgical resection of affected bowel.(8) If a diversion of the luminal contents was made to 'protect' the newly joined bowel then recurrent Crohn's disease did not occur beyond the join of the bowel. If however the diversion was reversed, undoing the protection of the joined bowel, then 40–60% of cases developed recurrent Crohn's disease within 6 months beyond the bowel join. Something in the luminal stream stimulated recurrence of Crohn's disease.

In general the outcome of Crohn's disease, evaluated over a long time interval, is only weakly predictable. Smoking and low educational levels were associated with more severe disease.[(9)] Crohn's disease is a continuum of disease whether mild, moderate or severe during which the same causative factors would be operative. Long-term disease factors would be worth relating to causation when finally established.

The luminal milieu of stomach, duodenum, jejunum, ileum, colon and anal region are all different. The observations of recurrent Crohn's disease after operation mentioned above, have been made with small bowel. One common factor is that at all levels of the gut microbes have a presence. Microbes are more plentiful in the distal small bowel and colon where Crohn's disease is found more frequently. Microbial factors in the environment need further consideration.

Microbial factors

Several observations in the microscopic pathology of tissues and also therapeutic responses to antibiotics in Crohn's disease point to microbes as being a central factor in the causation of Crohn's disease.

Firstly the microscopic pathology of Crohn's affected tissue in 60 to 70% of cases shows aggregates of epithelioid histiocytes often referred to as granulomata.[(10)] A number of bacteria, for instance *Mycobacterium tuberculosis, Yersinia, Chlamydia* and others, as well as foreign material, lead to the formation of granulomata. They are a non-specific guide to bacterial invasion but have a presence due to a variety of other non-bacterial causes as well.

The second line of observation implicating bacteria in Crohn's disease is that many cases of Crohn's disease respond to antibiotics, some in a spectacular manner.[(11)] Other cases of Crohn's disease do not respond to antibiotics at all. The conundrum of antibiotic response has not been unravelled but a microbial factor in the genesis of Crohn's disease would go some way.

Thirdly, in resected specimens of human bowel the draining lymph nodes of the bowel show a 28–48% presence of bacterial DNA.[(12)] Whether primacy of disease or secondary presence due to disease has not clearly been established for this observation. Similar studies for altered lymph nodes of the mesentery have been carried out in pigs[13] which were otherwise healthy: a considerable number of bacteria usually found in the gut lumen (*Campylobacter, Yersinia, Listeria or Salmonella*) were located in the mesenteric lymph nodes. Mesenteric lymph nodes are therefore a good marker of bacterial entry into the body.

A historical study in 1972[14] of small bowel bacteria in the distal small bowel and a replication in a very recent study in 2014[2], also of small intestinal bacteria, has not revealed a dominance of *Campylobacter, Yersinia, Listeria* or *Salmonella*. These studies excluded the clinical entity of bacterial overgrowth in the formation of Crohn's disease. The studies, 40 years apart, indicated that no huge progress on a causative microbe for Crohn's disease was made in this time period.

Viruses in Crohn's disease have received lesser attention. Even though rotavirus, norovirus and adeno-viruses may be found in the gastrointestinal tract, they were not found in Crohn's disease cases.[15]

Microbes have provided a fistful of hints but no concrete evidence of disease causation. The search for a bacterium causing Crohn's disease has been a challenge over the last 10–15 years. Four candidate bacteria have been advanced in this period (1) *Mycobacterium pseudotuberculosis*, (2) *Listeria*, (3) Enteroadhesive *E. Coli* and (4) *Mycoplasma*. These will be discussed in detail in the following chapters.

References

1. Corridoni D, Arseneau K, Cominelli F. Inflammatory bowel disease. Imm Letters 161:231–235 (2014)
2. Gevers D, Kugathasan S, Denson LA. The treatment-naïve microbiome in new-onset Crohn's disease. Cell Host and Microbe 15:382–392(2014)
3. Carriere J, Michaud A and Nguyen HT. Infectious etiopathogenesis of Crohn's disease. World J Gastroenterol 20:12102–12117 (2014)
4. Manichanh C, Borruel N, Casellas F et al. The gut microbiota in IBD. Nature Reviews Gastroenterol. Hepatol 9:599–608 (2012)
5. Jostins L, Ripke S, Weersma RK et al. Host-microbe interactions have shaped the genetic architecture of inflammatory bowel disease. Nature 491:119–124 (2012)
6. Goyette P, Boucher G, Mallon D et al. High-density mapping of the MHC identifies a shared role for HLA-DRBI 01:03 in inflammatory bowel diseases. Nature Genetics 47:172–181 (2015)
7. Kirsner's Inflammatory Bowel Disease 6th Ed. Eds Sartor RB and Sandborn WJ. Saunders Edinburgh (2004)

8. Rutgeerts P, Goboes K, Peeters M et al. Effect of faecal stream diversion on recurrence of Crohn's disease in the neoterminal ileum. Lancet 338:771–774 (1991)
9. Cosnes J, Bourrier A, Nion-Larmurier I et al. Factors affecting outcomes in Crohn's disease over 15 years. Gut: 61:1140–1145 (2012)
10. Riddell RH. Pathology of idiopathic inflammatory bowel disease pp. 399–424. In Kirsner's Inflammatory Bowel Disease. Eds Sartor B, Sanderson WJ. Ed Saunders (2004)
11. See Chapter 16
12. O'Brien CL, Pavli P, Gordon DM et al. Detection of bacterial DNA in lymph nodes of Crohn's disease patients using high throughput sequencing. Gut 63:1596–1606 (2014)
13. Mann E, Dzieciol M, Metzler-Zebeli BU et al. Microbiome of unreactive and pathologically altered ileocaecal lymph nodes of slaughter pigs. App Environ. Microbiol 80:193–203 (2014)
14. Vince A, Dyer NH, O'Grady FW et al. Bacteriological Studies in Crohn's disease. J Med Microbiol 5:219–229 (1972)
15. Wagner J, Sim WH, Lee KJ et al. Current knowledge and systematic review of viruses associated with Crohn's disease. Rev Med Virol 23:145–171 (2013)

-13-

Mycobacterium avium subspecies *paratuberculosis* (MAP)

OUTLINE: *Mycobacterium avium* subspecies *paratuberculosis* (MAP) have been implicated in a zoonosis, that is, spread of disease-causing bacteria from animal to man. In 1913 MAP were nominated as a causative organism but stainable MAP could not be found in Crohn's disease. MAP-disease in animals (Johne's disease) does not resemble human Crohn's disease. In 1968–1972 the proposals of 1913 re-emerged. DNA analysis for MAP provided the impetus but debates whether MAP caused Crohn's disease were always lost because of counter information.

MAP is the causative organism of an enteric infection in cattle, first described in 1895 by Johne and Frotheringham.[1] An analogous enteric infection occurs in sheep, goats, deer, rabbits and many other domestic animals. Johne's disease (JD) refers to an enteritis, hallmarked in cattle, by chronic diarrhoea, wasting and loss of thriftiness, and occasionally by loss of life. The chief diagnostic feature are the presence of stainable bacteria, known as 'acid fast bacilli' originally found in the submucosa of all affected animals.[1] Culturing MAP was described in 1912[2], but the process was unreliable and definition of JD by culture and serological testing has proved an issue since then with numerous subsequent reports in the literature providing improvement of diagnostic tests for the confirmation of JD in animals.

The first association of Crohn's disease (CD) in humans and Johne's disease in cattle was drawn by Dalziel in 1913[3] when he reported his ten cases of human disease which since then has tacitly been accepted as Crohn's disease. Dalziel reported that none of his ten cases revealed evidence of stainable acid fast bacilli, indicating that diagnostic criteria between JD and CD did not match. A further discrepancy between JD and CD is that mucosal ulceration, fissuring and fistula formation are

Table 12.1 Differences between Johne's disease and Crohn's disease

Feature	Johne's disease	Crohn's disease
Clinical manifestation	Enteritis. No mucosal ulcers or fissures	Mucosal ulcers or fissures present in all cases
Diagnosis	Acid-fast bacilli in 95% cases in submucosa	No acidfast bacilli
Prognosis	Chronic wasting, often non lethal	May be lethal if untreated

not found in JD[1] but are invariable manifestations of CD[4] (Table 12.1).

Casting the differences of 1895/1913 aside a new call emerged in 1968–1972[5,6] again drawing an analogy between JD and CD. Subsequent developments were notable for collaborations between gastroenterologists and microbiologists specializing in the detection of Mycobacteria. The means of laboratory evaluation now were diagnostic tests for bacterial DNA such as polymerase chain reaction (PCR) and in-situ hybridization for MAP in intestinal tissues. Many reports followed as listed by Quirke.[7] Of the 24 studies listed 15 studies failed to detect MAP by PCR in CD while in 9 reports detection varied between 5% to 100% of cases with CD. PCR detection of bacterial DNA is very sensitive and depends on the nature of DNA extraction from tissue and rigorous laboratory procedures requiring positive and negative controls at many points of the PCR process.

Microbiologists after 1980 maintained that MAP organisms were not stainable in Crohn's disease tissue because they existed as spores or spheroplasts.[8,9,10] Spore formation of *Mycobacterium tuberculosis* was put forward by Robert Koch in 1884[11] but has since then been considered unreliable information. Spores are considered non pathogenic and non stainable but if they germinate they become pathogenic, a cell wall develops and they again become stainable as acid fast bacilli.[12]

Professor F. Shanahan, an expert on IBD, has put forward 5 concerns and reasons why MAP are unlikely pathogens in CD.[13]

1. The epidemiology of CD/JD does not coincide
2. Poor sanitation, where mycobacteria would be abundant, appears to protect against CD
3. Immunosuppression worsens *Mycobacterium tuberculosis* but not CD
4. MAP detection in humans is not disease specific (also found in ulcerative colitis)
5. There is little serological evidence of MAP infestation in CD.

Two 'protagonist/antagonist' debates whether MAP is causative or not of CD have been published. One in 2001[14,15] and a further vigorous debate in 2011[16,17]. Outside observers can judge independently. The protagonists in both debates do not provide a convincing argument or winning formula.

In the publication *Is Crohn's Disease a Mycobacterial Disease?*[18] two polarized views are put strongly. Microbiologists state 'it is now conclusively and irrefutably shown that *MAP* can be found within the tissues of a major proportion of Crohn's disease patients' (R.J. Chiodini) while clinicians (D.Y. Graham) state 'definitive evidence of a mycobacterial agent specifically MAP, as critically involved in the pathogenesis of Crohn's disease is lacking.' Historical observations and modern observations indicate that MAP is not equatable with the causation of CD but may be, in some cases, a secondary invader of intestinal tissue involved with active Crohn's disease. The debate whether JD and CD are a zoonosis continues.[19]

References

1. Johne HA and Frothingham L. Ein eigenthumlicher Fall von Tuberkulose beim Rind. Dtsch Ztschr Tiermed Path 21:438–454 (1895)
2. Twort FW and Ingram GLY. A method for isolating and cultivating the Mycobacterium enteritides chronicae pseudotuberculosae bovis, Johne, and some experiments on the preparation of a diagnostic vaccine for pseudo-tuberculous enteritis of bovines. Proc Roy Soc Series B 84: 517–542 (1912)
3. Dalziel TK. Chronic interstitial enteritis. Br Med J ii:1068–1070 (1913)
4. Kirsner's Inflammatory Bowel Diseases. Eds RB Sartor and WJ Sandborn. Saunders, Edinburgh (2004)
5. Golde DW. Aetiology of regional enteritis. Lancet 291:1144–1145 (1968)
6. Patterson DSP and Allen WH. Chronic mycobacterial enteritis in ruminants as a model of Crohn's disease. Proc Roy Soc Med 65:998–1001 (1972)
7. Quirke P. Antagonist. Mycobacterium avium subspecies paratuberculosis as a cause of Crohn's disease. Gut 49:757–760 (2001)

8. Chiodini RJ, Van Kruiningen HJ, Thayer WR et al. Spheroplastic phase of mycobacteria isolated form patients with Crohn's disease. J Clin Microbiol 24:357–363 (1986)
9. Wall S, Kunze ZM, Saboor S et al. Identification of spheroplast-like agents isolated from tissues of patients with Crohn's disease and control tissues by polymerase chain reaction. J Clin Microbiol 31:1241–1245 (1993)
10. Kirsebom LA, Dasgupta S and Petterson BMF. Pleimorphism in Mycobacterium. Adv App Microbiol 80:81–112 (2012)
11. Gradmann C. Laboratory Disease. Robert Koch's Medical Bacteriology. pp. 77–78. The Johns Hopkins University Press Baltimore, (2009)
12. Lamont EA, Bannantine JP, Armien A et al. Identification and characterization of a spore-like morphotype in chronically starved *Mycobacterium* avium subsp. *Paratuberculosis* cultures. PLOS one 7:e30648 (2012)
13. Shanahan F, O'Mahoney J. The Mycobacteria story in Crohn's Disease. Am J Gastroenterol 100:1537–1538 (2005)
14. J Hermon Taylor. *Protagonist.* Mycobacterium avium subspecies paratuberculosis is a cause of Crohn's disease. 49:755–760 (2001)
15. Quirke P. *Antagonist.* Mycobacterium avium subspecies paratuberculosis is not a cause of Crohn's disease. Gut 49:755–760 (2001)
16. Van Kruiningen HJ. Where are the weapons of mass destruction – the *Mycobacterium paratuberculosis* in Crohn's disease. J Crohn's Colitis 5:638–644 (2011)
17. Chiodini RJ. The image of mass destruction inevitably leads to intellectual mass destruction. J Crohn's and Colitis 6:388–389 (2012)
18. Is Crohn's Disease a Mycobacterial Disease? Eds Mulder CJ and Tytgat GNJ. Kluwer Academic Press Dordrecht (1992)
19. Barkeha HW, Hendrick S, Debuck JM et al. Crohn's disease in Humans and Johne's in Cattle – Linked Diseases? In 'Zoonotic Pathogens in the Food Chain' Eds Krause D + Hendrick S. CABI (2010)

-14-

Enteric *Listeria monocytogenes* in Crohn's disease

OUTLINE: *Listeria monocytogenes* causes enteritis in sheep. The organism is stainable but has not been found in human Crohn's disease. Immune testing has found *Listeria* in human Crohn's disease. The suggestion is that *Listeria* may infect established Crohn's disease but are not causative of Crohn's disease. Further research is being conducted.

The organism *Listeria monocytogenes* which can cause severe disease in animals, was first described in rabbits in 1926[1] Fluid in the belly and enlarged mesenteric lymph nodes were noted but no changes in the gastrointestinal tract found then. A zoonosis, that is a disease of animals communicable to man, has been presumed for *Listeria monocytogenes* in Crohn's disease in the past but no direct evidence provided. Also arguing against a zoonosis is that *Listeria monocytogenes* is widely distributed in nature, found in soils, vegetables and foods.[2] It may be found in many animals and also in humans in a harmless form usually in the gastrointestinal tract where asymptomatic stool carriage occurs.[3] From a harmless commensal state it may become invasive and cause bacteremia or septicaemia. The reason for this transition has not been clarified even though *Listeria monocytogenes* provided an immunological/molecular model to microbiologists for defining the invasive 'profile' of bacteria.[4,5] Attributes for bacterial survival include its intracellular growth and ability to survive in cold climates and refrigeration. Despite the harmless nature of *Listeria monocytogenes*, it has been associated with acute attacks of gastroenteritis in humans.[6] In animals *Listeria monocytogenes* may cause severe gastroenteritis in sheep[7] and other ruminants[3] as well as colitis in horses.

Studies of *Listeria monocytogenes* in humans with Crohn's disease were not made until 1995. By using antibodies to *Listeria monocytogenes* and bacterial immune staining of Crohn's disease tissues, 75% of Crohn's disease cases were positively labelled with antibodies to *Listeria*.[(8)] The study which identified *Listeria monocytogenes* antibodies in Crohn's disease also included antibody detection to *E. Coli* and Streptococci which were also found in a high percentage of Crohn's disease cases leading to the conclusion that *Listeria monocytogenes* in Crohn's disease is probably a secondary invader.[(9)]

The potential of *Listeria monocytogenes* for being a causative factor of Crohn's disease received further attention. Listeria is a stainable organism that can be visualized histologically in enteric listeriosis of sheep[(7)] but has not been detected by microscopy in human Crohn's disease. Much more sensitive detection by bacterial DNA detection with nesting PCR has proved negative in all forms of Crohn's disease.[(10)] Another detailed immunohistochemical study in Crohn's disease, staining with appropriate antibodies for *Listeria monocytogenes*, proved negative.[(11)] In all studies appropriate control reactions were used and methodological error thereby excluded. A more recent analysis of culture of *Listeria monocytogenes* in Crohn's disease has shown a positive response in those cases of Crohn's disease with bacteremia or meningitis.[(12)] The study showed that Crohn's disease patients are more at risk of developing infection by *Listeria monocytogenes* than 'control' patients.

While the final verdict on *Listeria monocytogenes* in Crohn's disease is not in yet, all evidence indicates that *Listeria monocytogenes* is not causative of Crohn's disease but that super-infection with *Listeria monocytogenes* in Crohn's disease may occur, usually in the form of superimposed acute illness. Causation of Crohn's disease cannot be attributed to *Listeria monocytogenes*.

References

1. Murray EGD, Webb RA, Swann MBR. A disease of rabbits characterized by a large mononuclear leucocytosis, caused by a hitherto undescribed bacillus *Bacterium monocytogenes*. J Pathol Bacteriol 29:407–439 (1926)
2. Schleck WF, Lavigne PM, Bortolussi RD, et al. Epidemic listeriosis – evidence for transmission by food. NEJM 308:203–206 (1983)
3. Hoelzer K, Pouillo R and Dennis S. Animal models of Listeriosis: a comparative review of the current state of the art and lessons learned. Vet. Res 43: 1–27(2012)
4. Cossart P. Illuminating the landscape of host-pathogen interactions with the bacterium *Listeria monocytogens*. PNAS 108:19484–19491 (2011)

5. Hamon M, Bierne H and Cossart P. *Listeria monocytogenes*: a multifaceted model. Nature Reviews Microbiology 4:423–434 (2006)
6. Ooi ST and Lorber B. Gastroenteritis due to *Listeria* monocytogenes. Clin Infec Dis 40:1327–1337 (2005)
7. Fairley RA, Pasavento PA and Clark RG. *Listeria monocytogenes* infection of the alimentary tract (enteric listeriosis) of sheep in New Zealand. J. Comp. Path 146:308–313 (2012)
8. Liu Y, Van Kruiningen J, West AB et al. Immunocytochemical evidence *of Listeria, Escherichia Coli and Streptococcus* antigens in Crohn's disease. Gastroenterology 108: 1396–1404 (1995)
9. Brown WR. *Listeria*: The latest putative pathogenetic micro organism in Crohn's disease. Gastroenterology 108:1589–1590 (1995)
10. Chiba M, Fukushima T, Inoue Y et al. *Listeria monocytogenes* in Crohns disease. Scand J. Gastroenterol 33:430–434 (1998)
11. Walmsley RS, Anthony A, Sim R et al. Absence of *Escherichia coli, Listeria monocytogenes, and Klebsiella pneumoniae* antigens within inflammatory bowel disease tissues. J. Clin Pathol 51:657–661 (1998)
12. Miranda-Bautista J, Padilla-Suarez C, Bouza E. et al. *Listeria monocytogenes* infection in inflammatory bowel disease patients: case series and review of the literature. Eur J Gastroenterol 26:1247–1252 (2014)

-15-

Pathogenic *Escherichia coli* in Crohn's disease

OUTLINE: The organism *E. coli* is the most prolific and metabolically versatile of all known bacteria. A small number of harmful *E. coli* are known in humans and one variety that adheres to the bowel lining (AIEC) found to be most prolific in Crohn's disease. Antibody staining of the bacterium has confirmed the presence of *E. coli* now considered to be a secondary invader of established Crohn's disease.

The study of colonic bacteria was initially undertaken by Professor T. Escherich, and in his thesis of 1886 he described the *Bacterium coli commune* an organism now known as *Escherichia coli* or just *E. coli.*[1] It is a prolific bowel organism, and, metabolically as well as genetically, a most versatile organism which can grow with or without oxygen. It has the unusual genetic propensity of transferring its genetic pattern from one generation to the next or acquiring genetic material by lateral gene transfer. This transfers genetic material that translocates from one organism, either alive or dead, to another by transformation, transduction or conjugation[2] making the metabolic profile vary and potentially veering into the pathological variety. Most *E. coli* in the human colon are commensal (harmless) but several harmful pathological varieties of *E. coli* exist called pathovars, pathobionts or pathotypes. So far 8 pathotypes of *E. coli* have been discovered and described, the latest found in Germany in 2011 and known as Shiga toxin producing enteroaggregative *E. coli* (STEAEC)[3]. Each pathotype of *E. coli* has its own acronym and each of these pathotypes have an adhesion molecule specifically named. Some but not all pathotypes produce a toxin.

The interest in *E. coli* and its potential disguise into a pathotype has been a longstanding interest in Crohn's disease. In Crohn's disease *E. coli* are more prolific and they exhibit an adhesion index that is higher in Crohn's disease and ulcerative colitis compared to healthy control subjects.[4] This was a state of the art finding in the late 1980s.

The scene was set for further microbiological investigation along these lines in Crohn's disease. It was the French microbiologist Prof. A Darfeulle-Michaud who reported in 1998[5] that many ileal samples of Crohn's disease were colonized by a previously unappreciated class of *E. coli* named adherent invasive *E. coli* (AIEC). Much industry and much published work followed[6, 7, 8] with collaboration by both gastroenterologists and microbiologists. AIEC were found in enterocytes and macrophages of mesenteric lymph nodes in 21.7% of Crohn's disease versus 6.2% of control cases. The finding was that AIEC strains are associated specifically with the ileal mucosa of Crohn's disease.[6] One productive outreach was that AIEC organisms could be taken to experimental animals there to define their molecular and immunological characteristics. Two recent attributes of AIEC have been shown in mice. Firstly that Western diet[9] may induce a dysbiosis (altered microbial composition of beneficial and harmful bacteria) and proliferation of AIEC or AIEC may alter microbial composition in genetically engineered mice[10] and thereby induce colitis. Undoubtedly AIEC has moved to the centre stage of the disease process of Crohn's disease.

As so often occurs in the science of human disease opposite findings were soon reported. Histological and antibody staining for *E. coli* showed no preponderance of *E. coli* in inflammatory bowel disease though the pathotype AIEC was not specifically detected by those studies.[11] A study using similar methodology and similar actions was reported several years thereafter.[12]

The final conclusions on AIEC in Crohn's disease are not yet in. As so often with nominated organisms, for example *MAP* or *Listeria monocytogenes*, the final hard proof is difficult to come by. The place of AIEC most probably is that of a secondary invader nevertheless it is worthwhile keeping an open mind and to conduct further studies in humans rather than genetically engineered animals.

References

1. Grove DI. Tapeworms, lice and prions. pp. 339–347 Oxford University Press, Oxford, (2014)
2. O'Malley M.A. Philosophy of Microbiology pp. 65–94 Cambridge University Press, Cambridge, (2011)

3. Clements A, Young JC, Constantinou N. et al. Infection strategies of enteric pathogenic *Escherichia coli*. Gut Microbes 3:71–87 (2012)
4. Burke DA and Axon ATR. Adhesive *Escherichia coli* in inflammatory bowel disease and infective diarrhoea. Br. Med. J. 297:102–104 (1988)
5. Darfeuille-Michaud A, Neut C, Barnich N et al. Presence of adherent *Escherichia coli* strains in ileal mucosa of patients with Crohn's disease. Gastroenterol. 115:1405–1413 (1998)
6. Darfeuille-Michaud A, Boudeau J, Bulois P et al. High prevalence of adherent-invasive *Escherichia coli* associated with ileal mucosa in Crohn's disease. Gastroenterol 127:412–421 (2004)
7. Rolhion N and Darfeuille-Michaud A. Adherent-invasive *Escherichia coli* in inflammatory bowel disease. Inflamm Bowel Dis 13:1277–1283 (2007)
8. Carriere J, Darfeuille-Michaud A, Nguyen HTT. Infectious etiopathogenesis of Crohn's disease. World J Gastroenterol 14:12102–12117 (2008)
9. Martinez-Medina M, Denizot J, Dreux N et al. Western diet induces dysbiosis with increased *E. Coli* in CEABAC 10 mice, alters host barrier function favouring AIEC colonisation. Gut 63:113–124 (2014)
10. Chaissaing B, Koren O, Carvalho FA et al. AIEC pathobiont instigates chronic colitis in susceptible hosts by altering microbiota composition. Gut 63:1069–1080 (2014)
11. Walmsley RS, Anthony A, Sim R et al. Absence of *Escherichia coli, Listeria monocytogenes* and *Klebsiella pneumoniae* antigens within inflammatory bowel disease tissues. J. Clin Pathol 51:567–661 (1998)
12. Magin WS, Van Kruiningen HJ, Colombel JF. Immunohistochemical search for viral and bacterial antigens in Crohn's disease. J. Crohns Colitis 7:161–166 (2013)

-16-

Mycoplasma in the causation of Crohn's disease

OUTLINE: Mollicutes are the smallest known bacteria which are difficult to locate by microscope or grow in culture. *Mycoplasma* are a subgenus of mollicutes and four species of mycoplasmas cause disease in humans. Generally *Mycoplasma* grow on surface lining cells of organs and cause chronic disease. *Mycoplasma fermentans* causes oral and genital ulceration as well as arthritis, all occurring in Crohn's disease. Five different scientific approaches support the presence of *M. fermentans* in Crohn's disease. The phase of infection fall into acute infective stage and a chronic antigenic phase that can last more than two years. Antibiotics may eradicate *M. fermentans* in the acute infective stage. Many other bacterial characteristics support a causative role for *M. fermentans* in Crohn's disease.

The previous three chapters have highlighted the scientific ingenuity employed to find a causative organism for Crohn's disease. The shadows of an organism never produced a concrete body with which the disease process of Crohn's disease could be associated. Any new scientific investigation would need to correlate clinical expression of the disease with an organism to provide a key to the road ahead. *Mollicutes* seemed a worthy group for scrutiny to provide such a path.

Mollicutes are so called because these organisms have a single layered limiting membrane rather than a double layered lipid cell wall. Hence the name 'mollis' for soft and 'cutis' for skin: a malleable soft skin. *Mollicutes* were first observed by Nocard and others in 1898[1] from cases of pleuropneumonia in cattle. These organisms passed through bacterial filters and, unlike viruses, could be cultured. They were initially designated as viruses but then reports between 1920 and 1950+ led them to be known as PPLOs (pleuropneumonia-like organisms) after Nocard's original findings. The term PPLO was applied to numerous isolates from many sources until in 1956 when a reclassification of PPLOs into genus and species took place.[2] Several subsequent subdivisions and realignments have occurred.[3,4,5] The mollicutes constitute eight genera one of which is '*Mycoplasma*'. In the genus '*Mycoplasma*' over 200 species have been recorded mostly in animals, plants, fishes, insects and some in humans. In humans 16 species of *Mycoplasma* were recorded by 2002 of which 4 were considered pathogenic and the others commensals[6] (Table 16.1).

Mycoplasma have attracted a notoriety particularly for a long history of incorrect assignment to diseases. For example *M. fermentans* has been associated with fibromyalgia, HIV, chronic fatigue syndrome, Gulf War syndrome and arthritis. All but the last disease association have been rejected and the causation of arthritis is still under consideration. Many mycoplasmas have had a long lead up time before a clinical association was made. *Mycoplasma pneumoniae* was first recorded by Eaton in 1944 but only formally recognised as causing pneumonia in 1962[7]. The mycoplasma of urethritis[8] reported in 1953 had to wait until 1981 before correctly being isolated as *Mycoplasma genitalium*.[9] Over 50 years many revised reports on *Mycoplasma* have appeared. All these precedents have provided a daunting setting in trying to find a mycoplasma associated with Crohn's disease. For Crohn's disease the spotlight fell on *Mycoplasma*, either of the pathogenic or commensal variety, for the following reasons:

1. Mycoplasmas are usually associated with subclinical, subtle, slowly progressive or chronic disease.
2. Mycoplasmas are not readily detectable by light microscopy using conventional staining methods but can be shown by dark field illumination[10] and other special stain techniques.
3. Mycoplasmas are difficult to grow in culture and require specific conditions for culture for which reason *Mycoplasma* in Crohn's disease may not have been found in the past.
4. In humans mycoplasmas, both pathogenic or commensal, are found in the oropharynx[11] and anal canal.[8] From the oral cavity they might proceed to the gastrointestinal tract as a potential pathogen. Certainly in the gastrointestinal tract of pigs mycoplasmas are found[12] and also in the mesenteric lymph nodes[13] of pigs with gastrointestinal inflammation.

A zoonosis is not implied but the precedent of *Mycoplasma* in the gastrointestinal tract has been set.

5. Mycoplasmas are usually found on epithelial linings or surfaces, both in humans and animals where they cause disease (Table 16.1). The likelihood of mycoplasma causing disease in the epithelium of the gastrointestinal tract therefore seemed a possibility.

Table 16.1 – Association of *Mycoplasma*, epithelia of organs and disease formation

Organ/epithelium	Organism	Disease
Broncho/alveolar	*M. pneumoniae*	Pneumonia (humans)
Mammary epithelium	*M. agalactia*	Mastitis (animals, assumed for humans)
Uro-epithelium	*M. genitalium*	Urethritis (humans)
Reproductive organs	*M. hominis*	Pelvic Inflammatory Disease (humans)
Synovial epithelium	*M. fermentans*	Arthritis (humans)
Gastrointestinal epithelia	???	?? Crohn's disease

Mycoplasma in Crohn's disease

A lead into a possible association of *Mycoplasma* with Crohn's disease was obtained from a historical review of 1948–1953 of *Mycoplasma* (then called PPLO) that caused disease in humans. *Mycoplasmas* were reported in oral ulceration,[14] penile[15] and vaginal[16] ulceration. All these are sites where Crohn's disease may manifest with ulceration. The typing of genitourinary mycoplasmas has been a confusing one but now resolved (Table 16.1) into *Mycoplasma hominis* for pelvic inflammation in women and *Mycoplasma genitalium* causing urethritis. The observation of *Mycoplasma fermentans* in penile ulceration[15] is now considered the first reported case of *Mycoplasma fermentans*, an organism whose role in genital ulceration has not been sustained[17] and mostly *Mycoplasma fermentans* attributed to causing arthritis[18] but even this attribution is conjectural. The historical case of oral ulceration[14] could have been *Mycoplasma orale* which genetically is closely allied to *Mycoplasma fermentans*[19] frequently found in the oropharynx confined to oral ulcers.[20, 21, 22] Thus in the historical reports oral and genital ulceration could be linked to *Mycoplasma fermentans*, while oral/genital ulceration is found in Crohn's disease. At least 34% of newly diagnosed cases of Crohn's disease also have arthritis.[23] A potential link of *Mycoplasma fermentans* with Crohn's disease seemed possible.

A signature case of *Mycoplasma fermentans* in Crohn's disease

Due to personal publications concerning *Mycoplasma* in Crohn's disease[24, 25] a young patient who had searched the electronic libraries and repositories of information phoned me to let me know she had Crohn's disease as well as *Mycoplasma fermentans* found on her. She indeed had a procto-colectomy for Crohn's disease and was now troubled by chronic fatigue which led her physician, Professor R. Philpott, an Infectious diseases physician, to search for *Mycoplasma fermentans*. Blood and tissue samples from resected bowel with ulcers were sent separately to two laboratories for PCR analysis of *Mycoplasma fermentans*. Both laboratories (Mrs J. Burke, Australian Biologics, Sydney and Dept. of Veterinary Pathology, Melbourne) reported a strong presence of *Mycoplasma fermentans* in resected tissues. Subsequent analysis of tonsillar tissue, removed for tonsillitis after the procto-colectomy, again revealed *Mycoplasma fermentans* on PCR analysis. After prolonged treatment with antibiotics, a complete recovery from chronic fatigue was made. No further manifestations of Crohn's disease have since occurred.

The above case in the light of preceding comments on *Mycoplasma* and Crohn's disease led to a prospective search for *Mycoplasma fermentans* in Crohn's disease utilizing four analytic approaches.

1. Cytoplasmic DNA staining for organisms
2. PCR analysis for *Mycoplasma fermentans* in colonic ulcers of cases deemed to have Crohn's disease.
3. Immune staining of lipopeptide of *Mycoplasma fermentans* in Crohn's disease
4. Observed responses to antibiotics in acute cases of Crohn's disease where *M. fermentans* was detected.

1. Cellular DNA staining for *Mycoplasma*

Mycoplasmas often infect tissue cultures. In order to detect infective *Mycoplasma* in cell culture a fluorescent dye specific for DNA is generally used.[26,27] This effective method to detect *Mycoplasma* was employed on fresh tissue obtained at operation for Crohn's disease, fixed in alcohol and sections viewed with a fluorescent microscope. Only in Crohn's cases, but not control cases, could intra-epithelial DNA in the cytoplasm be demonstrated (Fig. 16.1). The intracellular DNA was patchy often located to a group of crypt cells. No species identification of *Mycoplasma* can be attributed to this test but at least intracellular organisms could be readily demonstrated in Crohn's disease.

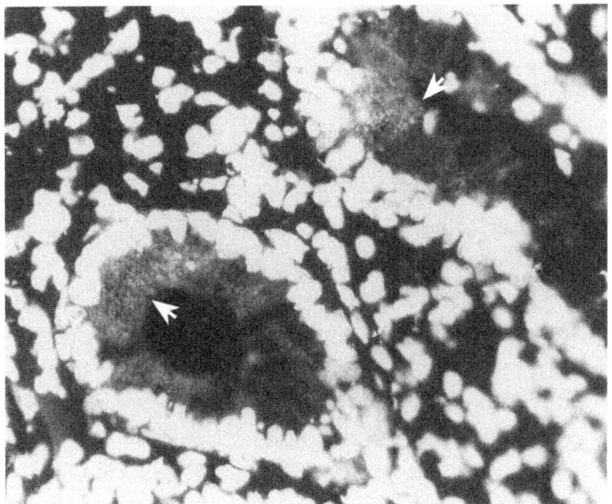

Figure 16.1 Fluorescent staining for DNA in acute Crohn's disease. Positive stipulation for DNA in the cytoplasm of small bowel epithelial cells reflects presence of bacteria not seen in healthy control cases.

2. Polymerase chain reaction for *Mycoplasma fermentans* DNA in tissue

Tissue samples were obtained from acute and chronic Crohn's disease and the DNA extracted by standard methods. Nucleotide primers for *Mycoplasma fermentans* were selected according to Wang[28] and

Hawkins[29] and amplification of these primers carried out according to standard methods with TAQ polymerase. The amplified DNA product was removed and detected by gel electrophoresis (Fig. 16.2) stained with ethidium bromide and viewed by UV light. The sequence of amplified DNA was compared with DNA sequences of *Mycoplasma fermentans* and found to be that of *Mycoplasma fermantans*. In 9 cases of acute Crohn's disease, *Mycoplasma fermentans* was detected and a further two cases were negative for *Mycoplasma fermentans*. These two cases had chronic longstanding Crohn's disease for more than 5 years. No control cases (healthy colonic tissue collected at colonoscopy) showed a positive PCR for *Mycoplasma* fermentans.

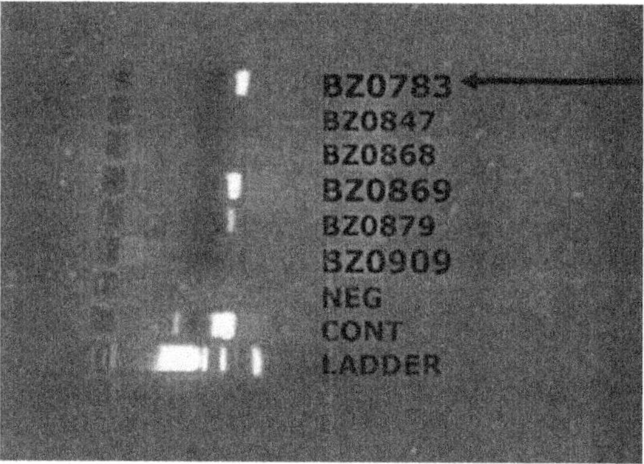

Figure 16.2 Gel electrophoresis of PCR for *Mycoplasma fermentans* (top two rows) of biopsies from Crohn's disease with 'controls' and 'molecular ladder'.

3. *Mycoplasma fermentans* lipopeptide detection in Crohn's disease

Immunostaining for lipopeptide of *Mycoplasma fermentans* was undertaken with mouse monoclonal antibodies[30] kindly donated by Prof. K. Wise, Department of Molecular Microbiology, University of Missouri, School of Medicine USA. Detection of antibody reaction was with hydrogen peroxide and diaminobenzidine tetrachloride, a standard detection method. Neutrophils stained strongly positive for lipopeptide in addition to weaker staining of fibroblasts. Only two cases of chronic Crohn's disease were studied due to limited supply of antibody. (Fig. 16.3)

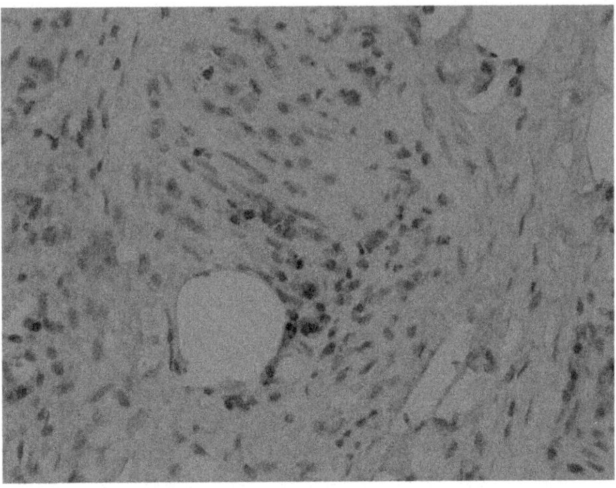

Figure 16.3 Mouse monoclonal antibody staining for lipopeptide of *Mycoplasma fermentans* (brown stain) in chronic Crohn's disease, not found in control cases. Immune cells positive amongst tissue fibrosis.

4. Antibiotic response to clarithromycin

Clarithromycin is a macrolide antibiotic readily absorbed via the oral route and concentrated in macrophages[31, 32] which may be prominent in Crohn's disease. All nine acute cases of Crohn's disease resolved completely with antibiotics and without further recurrence (after 3 years) after a six weeks course of antibiotic.

Antibiotic use in chronic Crohn's disease with stricturing was used on one case that did not undergo operation. Healing of ileal ulcers but not resolution of stricturing (Fig. 16.4) occurred. No further need for operation arose.

Clarithromycin was used for two 6 week periods after ileo-colonic resection for chronic Crohn's disease. None of 14 cases operated upon developed recurrent Crohn's disease where this might be expected to occur in 50% of untreated cases.

A number of avenues of research just outlined and the historical perspective make *Mycoplasma fermentans* a plausible organism in the causation of Crohn's disease. However to date causality has not definitely been proven nevertheless warrants further consideration.

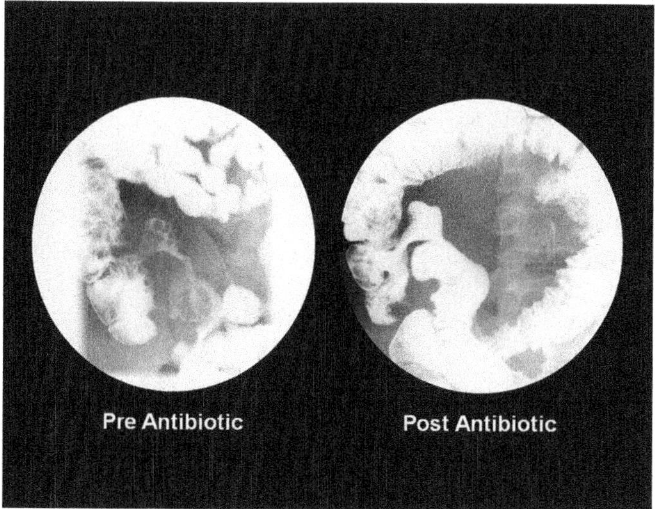

Figure 16.4 X-rays, with contrast, of distal small bowel showing narrowing and ulceration before antibiotic treatment and healing of ulcers after a course of antibiotics but no change of fibrosis.

Other Features of *Mycoplasma fermentans* in Crohn's disease

Several aspects of *Mycoplasma fermentans* in humans need commentary in the light of the findings outlined above.

Mycoplasma has a strong association with the oral cavity in health and disease. In health *Mycoplasma fermentans* can be found in saliva in between 44%(22) and 54.7%(21) of healthy subjects, mainly in young children. A lesser percentage of Mycoplasma was found in saliva in a worldwide analysis of cases.(33) In pathological conditions such as tonsillitis(34) and gingivitis(35) Mycoplasmal DNA is frequently found but not subtyped for *Mycoplasma fermentans*. In Crohn's disease antibiotics in children are significantly more often used for oropharyngeal infections(36) than cases of ulcerative colitis or the control population.(37,38) The relevance of an oral source for an organism causing infection in the gastrointestinal tract is possible but needs further scrutiny in Crohn's disease.

Antigens that drive immune stimulation in Crohn's disease have to date not been defined. Antibody staining of lipopeptide derived from *Mycoplasma fermentans* suggest that this lipopeptide could be a likely antigen for the chronic inflammatory response in Crohn's disease. Wise[30] and Muhlradt[39,40] highlighted the profound immuno-stimulation of mycoplasmal lipopeptide, in excess of that of bacterial lipopolysaccharide,[41] produced in tissues. The synthetic derivative of the lipopeptide of *Mycoplasma fermentans* induces macrophage proliferation, maturation of dendritic cells and promotes release of nitric oxide, tumour necrosing factor (TNF) and prostaglandins from tissues.[39, 42, 43] All of these are components of the inflammatory response in Crohn's disease.

The complete genomic sequence of *Mycoplasma fermentans* has been established[44] which highlights that much of the gene sequence regulates transport properties and protein components particularly those of lipopeptide of the limiting membrane of *Mycoplasma*. Changes in the protein of the lipoprotein determines immunogenicity[45] and may account for the different strains of *Mycoplasma fermentans*. It is possible that strain expression may have an impact on disease expression caused by *Mycoplasma fermentans*.

Mycoplasmas in humans have a disquieting relationship to cigarette smoking. In the presence of smoking *Mycoplasma pneumoniae* cannot be eradicated in chest infections. Likewise smoking prevents improvement and healing of Crohn's disease. Does the connectivity of smoking in Crohn's disease/pneumonia support a role for a mycoplasma in Crohn's disease? How would this come about? One study[46] suggests that smoking prevents clearance of bacteria from macrophages, a mechanism that may operate in *Mycoplasma pneumoniae* and *Mycoplasma fermentans* in Crohn's disease.

The phases of infection by *Mycoplasma fermentans* so far observed in Crohn's disease seem to fall into two varieties (Fig. 16.5 and Fig. 16.6). The first is an active infective phase that produces mild symptoms and an organism that appears sensitive to antibiotics followed by a chronic antigenic phase which produces more severe symptoms, fibrosis and a disease pattern that does not respond to antibiotics. Chronicity of tissue reaction and long term retention of bacterial antigens has been shown with several other bacteria, for example *Coxiella burnetti*.[47, 48] *Mycoplasma* may also be retained in tissue for a long time and may not be readily cleared.[49] These bacterial characteristics may play a part in the development of Crohn's disease.

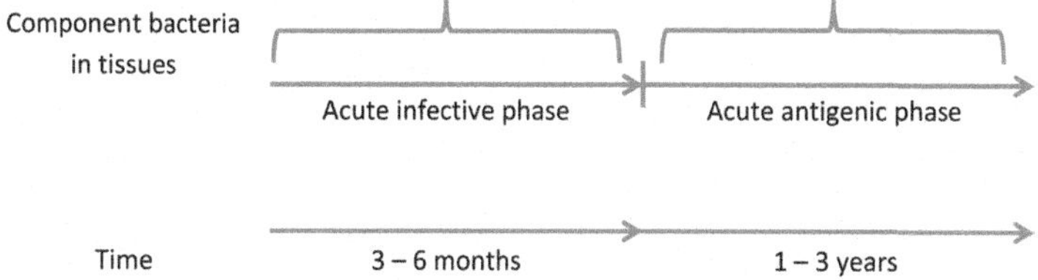

Figure 16.5 Phases of *Mycoplasma fermentans* involvement of bowel tissue in the course of time.

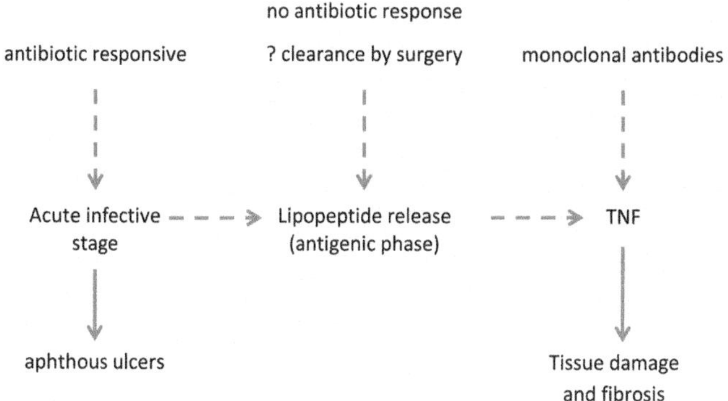

Figure 16.6 Therapies of value in the treatment of *Mycoplasma fermentans* over the course of time.

Finding evidence of a specific organism in Crohn's disease by molecular DNA raises the question of a causative or an opportunistic organism. An association does not prove causation and there has always remained a thin line between gut commensals and pathogens.(50) Ideally Koch's postulate need to be fulfilled but attempts to transmit *Mycoplasma fermentans* as early as 1952(13) failed to reproduce a disease process in humans. Molecular guidelines have been defined to establishing microbial disease causation(51, 52) in place of the classical Koch's postulates. These guidelines would be pertinent to follow as *Mycoplasma fermentans* is extremely difficult to culture.

Conclusions

In conclusion *Mycoplasma fermentans* better than any other organism accounts for the symptomatology of Crohn's disease. Use and response to antibiotics do not favour a secondary infection. Certainly the confirmation that pathological events with *Mycoplasma* are central to Crohn's disease far outweighs the lack of confirmation that MAP, *Listeria monocytogenes* or pathogenic *E. coli* provide for a disease process in Crohn's disease. A search in the use of antibiotics for Crohn's disease may provide further clues, as discussed in the next chapter.

References

1. Nocard E, Roux E, Borrel M et al. Microbe de la peripneumonie. Ann Inst Pasteur (Paris) 12:240–262 (1898)
2. Edward DG and Freundt EA. The classification and nomenclature of organisms of the pleuropneumonia group. J. Gen. Microbiol 14:197–207(1956)
3. Neimark HC. Division of Mycoplasmas into subgroups. J. Gen. Microbiol 63:249–263 (1971)
4. Weisburg WG, Tully JG, Rose DL et al. A Phylogenetic analysis of the Mycoplasmas: Basis for their classification. J. Baceteriol 171:6455–6467 (1989)
5. Stakenborg T, Vicca J, Verhelst R et al. Evaluation of tRNA gene PCR for identification of mollicutes. J. Clin Microbiol 43:4558–4566 (2005)
6. Blanchard A and Bebear CM. Mycoplasmas of humans pp. 45–71 in 'Molecular Biology and Pathogenicity of Mycoplasmas' Eds S. Razin and R. Herrmann. Kluwer Academic/Plenum Publishers, New York (2002)
7. Marmion BP. Eaton Agent – science and scientific acceptance: a historical commentary. Revs Infect Dis 12:338–353 (1990)
8. Nicol CS and Edward DG. Role of organisms of the pleuropneumonia group in human genital infections. Br J Ven Dis 92:141–150 (1953)
9. Taylor-Robinosn D. The history and role of *Mycoplasma genitalium* in sexually transmitted diseases. Genitourin Med 71:1–8 (1995)
10. Barnard JE and Smiles J. Contributions to the study of the filterable viruses. B. Morphology of bovine pleuropneumonia. J. Royal Mic Soc 46:253–264(1926)
11. Tully JG. Current status of the mollicute flora of humans. Clin Infect Dis 17 (Suppl 1) 52–9 (1993)
12. Gourlay RN, Wyld SG and Leach RH. Mycoplasma sualvi, a new species from the intestinal and urogenital tracts of pigs. Int J System Bacteriol 28:289–292 (1978)
13. Mann E, Dzieciol M, Metzer-Zebev BU et al. Microbiome of unreactive and pathologically altered ileocaecal lymph nodes of slaughter pigs. App. Environ Microbiol. 80:193–203 (2014)
14. Melczer N. Zur aetiologie und pathogenese der Vincent'schen angina und der stomatitis ulceromembranosa. Dermatologica 94:13–24 (1947)
15. Ruiter M and Wentholt MD. The occurrence of a pleuropneumonia-like organism in fuso-spirillary infections of the human genital mucosa. J. Invest Dermatol 18:313–325 (1952)
16. Ruiter M, Wentholt MM. Isolation of a pleuropneumonia-like organism (G-strain) in a case of fusospirillary vulvovaginitis. Acta Derm Venereol 33:123–129 (1953)

17. Deguchi T, Gilroy CB and Taylor-Robinson D. Failure to detect *Mycoplasma fermentans*, *Mycoplasma penetrans* or *Mycoplasma pirum* in the urethra of patients with nongonococcal urethritis. Eur J. Clin Microbiol Infect Dis 15:169–171 (1996)
18. Horowitz S, Evinson B, Borer A et al. *Mycoplasma fermentans* in rheumatoid arthritis and other inflammatory arthritides. J. Rheumatol 27:2747–2753 (2000)
19. Ditty SE, Li B, Zhang S et al. Characterisation of an IS element in *Mycoplasma orale* that is highly homologous to M. *fermentans*. Curr Microbiol 46:302–06 (2003)
20. Zouboulis C, Turnbull JR and Muhlradt PF. High seroprevalance of anti *Mycoplasma fermentans* antibiodies in patients with malignant aphthosis J. Invest Dermatol 121:211–212 (2003)
21. Shibata K, Kaga M, Kudo M et al. Detection of *Mycoplasma fermentans* in saliva sampled from infants, preschool and school children, adolescents and adults by a polymerase reaction-based assay. Microbiol Immunol 43:521–525 (1999)
22. Chingbingyong MI, Hughes CV. Detection of *Mycoplasma fermentans* in human saliva with a polymerase chain reaction-based assay. Arch Oral Biol 41:311–314 (1996)
23. Orchard TR, Wordsworth BP and Jewell DP. Peripheral arthropathies in inflammatory bowel disease: their articular distribution and natural history. Gut 42:387–391 (1998)
24. Roediger WEW and Macfarlane GT. A role for intestinal mycoplasmas in the aetiology of Crohn's disease? J Appl Microbiol 92:377–81 (2002)
25. Roediger WEW. Intestinal mycoplasma in Crohn's disease. Novartis Found Symp 263:85–98 (2004)
26. Chen TR. In situ detection of mycoplasma contamination in cell culture by fluorescent Hoechst 33258 stain. Exp Cell Res 104:255–262 (1977)
27. Pjura PE, Grezeskowiak K, Dickerson RE. Binding of Hoechst 33258 to the minor groove of Ɖ-DNA. J. Mol Biol 197:257–271 (1987)
28. Wang RYH, Hu WS, Dawson MS et al. Selective detection of *Mycoplasma fermentans* by polymerase chain reaction and by using a nucleotide sequence within the insertion sequence-like element. J. Clin Microbiol 30:245–248 (1992)
29. Hawkins RE, Rickman LS, Vermund SD et al. Association of Mycoplasma and human immunodeficiency virus infection: detection of amplified *Mycoplasma fermentans* DNA in blood. J Infect Dis 165:581–585 (1992)
30. Wise KS, Theiss PM and Lo SC. A family of strain-variant surface lipoproteins of Mycoplasma fermentans. Infect Immun. 61:3327–3333 (1993)
31. Subramanian S, Roberts CL. Hart A. et al. Replication of colonic Crohn's disease mucosal *Escherichia coli* isolates within macrophages and their susceptibility to antibiotics. Antimicrob Agents Chemo 52:427–434 (2008)
32. Cai M, Bonella F, Dai H et al. Macrolides inhibit cytokine production by alveolar macrophages in bronchiolitis obliterans organizing pneumonia. Immunobiology 218:930–937 (2013)
33. Nasidze I, Li J, Quinque D et al. Global diversity in the human salivary microbiome. Genome Research 19:636–643 (2009)
34. Esposito S, Marchisio P, Capaccio P et al. Role of atypical bacteria in children undergoing tonsillectomy because of severely recurrent acute tonsillopharyngitis. Eur J. Clin. Microbiol Infect Dis 27:1233–37 (2008)

35. Holt RD, Wilson M and Musa S. Mycoplasmas in plaque and saliva of children and their relationship to gingivitis. J. Periodontal 66:97–101 (1995)
36. Wurzelman JI, Lyles CM and Sandler RS. Childhood infections and the risk of inflammatory bowel disease. Dig Dis Sci 39:550–560 (1994)
37. Hviid A, Svanstrom H and Frisch M. Antibiotic use and inflammatory bowel disease in childhood. Gut 60:49–54 (2011)
38. Virta L, Auvinen A, Helenius H et al. Association of repeated exposure to anitibiotics with the development t of pediatric Crohn's disease – A Nationwide register-based Finnish control study. Am J Epidemiol 175:775–784 (2012)
39. Muhlradt PF and Frisch M. Purification and partial biochemical characterization of a *Mycoplasma fermentans*-derived substance that activates macrophages to release nitric oxide, TNF, and IL-6. Infect Immun 62:3801–3807 (1994)
40. Muhlradt PF, Kiess M, Meyer H et al. Isolation, structure elucidation and synthesis of a macrophage stimulatory lipopeptide from *Mycoplasma fermentans* acting at picomolar concentration. J Exp Med 185:1951–58 (1997)
41. Galanos C, Gumenscheimer M, Muhlradt P et al. MALP-2, a Mycoplasma lipopeptide with classical endotoxic properties: end of an era of LPS monopoly? J. Endotoxin Res 6:471–6 (2000)
42. Kaufman A, Muhlradt PF, Gemsa D. et al. Induction of cytokines and chemokines in human monocytes by *Mycolasma* fermentans-derived lipoprotein MALP-2. Infect Immun 67:6303–8 (1999)
43. Weigt H, Muhlradt PF, Emmendorffer A. et al. Synthetic mycoplasma-derived lipopeptide MALP-2 induces maturation and function of dendritic cells. Immunobiol 207:223–233 (2003)
44. Rechnitzer H, Brzuszkiewicz E, Strittmatter A. et al. Genome features and insights into the biology of *Mycoplasma fermentans*. Microbiology 157:760–773 (2011)
45. Chambaud I, Wroblewski H and Blanchard A. Interactions between mycoplasma lipoproteins and the host system. Trends Microbiol 7:493–499 (1999)
46. Baqir M, Chen C-Z, Martin RJ et al. Cigarette smoke decreases MARCO expression in macrophages: implication in *Mycoplasma pneumoniae* infection. Resp Med 107:1604–1610 (2008)
47. Marmion BP, Storm PA, Ayres JG et al. Long term persistence of *Coxiella burnetii* after acute primary infection. Q J Med 98:7–20 (2005)
48. Sukocheva OA, Marmion BP, Storm PA et al. Long term persistence after acute Q fever of non-infective *Coxiella brunetii* cell components including antigens. Q J Med 103:847–863 (2010)
49. Taylor-Robinson D and Behnke J. The prolonged persistence of mycoplasmas in culture. J Med Microbiol 23:89–92 (1987)
50. Gilmore MS and Ferreti JJ. The thin line between gut commensal and pathogen. Science 299:1999–2000 (2003)
51. Fredericks D and Relman DA. Sequence-based identification of microbial pathogens: a reconsideration of Koch's postulates. Clin Microbiol Rev 9:18–33 (1996)
52. Ferreira RBR, Willing BP and Finlay BB. Bringing Koch's postulates to the table in IBD. Cell Host Microbe 9:353–354 (2011)

-17-

Antibiotics in Crohn's disease: any clues?

OUTLINE: Antibiotics are used in Crohn's disease when there is bodily invasion of bacteria from ulcers in Crohn's lesions. Non septic cases of Crohn's disease may sometimes respond to antibiotics in a spectacular way. The type of bacterium and the phase of bacterial invasion appear critical to an antibiotic response in Crohn's disease.

Antibiotics have since the 1970's been used as a therapeutic option in the treatment of CD. While the septic and perianal complications of CD undoubtedly require antibiotics their use in non septic CD remains questionable because consistent scientific evidence of usefulness is lacking and because of a lack of knowledge of a precise organism to treat in CD. Where antibiotics do aid acute CD some inferences on causation may be drawn. Quite separately has emerged that repeated exposure to oral antibiotics in childhood has led to a predisposition of developing CD later in life.

Supposition that atypical Mycobacteria (MAP) might cause CD provided a platform for the use of long term antibiotics in the treatment of CD. Following an open label trial of clarithromycin, rifabutin and clofazimine which appeared successful, a two year randomized control study was initiated in Australia.(1) This Australian trial was also preceded by a non randomized study, with rifabutin and clarithromycin at St George's Hospital London(2) which did reveal improvement of CD. The Australian study by Selby et al.(1) concluded that long term use of antibiotics in CD did not provide evidence of sustained clinical benefit and as editorialized in the prestigious journal of 'Gastroenterology', the Australian trial did not support a role for MAP in the causation of CD.(3) With a modern scientific quirkiness of 'subset analysis' it emerged in the Australian trial that those cases of CD that did respond to antibiotics, remained in remission[4] whereas non-antibiotic responders relapsed. A scientific example of the 'good and the bad' with regard to conclusions of trials. A similar scenario regarding response to antibiotics was repeated in the UK (Liverpool) with the use of clarithromycin as a single antibiotic, that is, monotherapy. The initial open label study[5] concluded that an impressive response to clarithromycin occurred in a group of CD patients who had been resistant to other therapy. Subsequently a randomized control trial showed that clarithromycin (1 g for 12 weeks) was ineffective in active CD.[6] Again a subset analysis of responding patients did show improvement and remission. Results in Australia and the UK seemed mirror images of each other. In spite of these two reports when results of sixteen different trials were drawn together[7] the conclusion arose that use of nitroimidazole or clofazimine appears to be effective in patients with CD. As recently as 2013 these conclusions were upheld.[8]

In general there is some clinical improvement to be got from antibiotic treatment in CD but the 'why' and the 'when' appears not to be answered. Criticisms of antibiotic trials include the following.

1. Response of CD to antibiotics is judged on 'Disease activity Index' an index that does not correlate to bacterial groups, that is commensals, conditional pathogens or pathogens which have not been measured before and after treatment.
2. The target organism for antibiotic treatment has not been clearly defined though mycobacteria (MAP) were nominated in earlier studies but their presence could not be quantitatively measured. Later studies nominated pathogenic *E. coli* and again these were not cultured before and after treatment.
3. The phases of bacterial causation of CD may fall into an 'infective phase' or an 'antigenic phase' (see Chapter 16). Do both phases respond equally to antibiotics? This question remains unanswered.
4. Do long term use of antibiotics, that is for more than 10 weeks, induce resistance in any putative pathogenic organism?

Given the above reservations and bacterial analyses of the previous chapters (13–16), a re-examination of how antibiotics could be used in acute CD was done. Cases that demonstrated an acute CD-like ulcer/s or following ileo-colonic resection were treated with short term clarithromycin (500 mg twice a day for six weeks) as outlined in the previous chapter. The premise, whether correct or incorrect, was that *Mycoplasma fermentans* underlay the disease process. This organism may develop resistance to long term antibiotic exposure.[9] All acute CD patients were tested for *Mycoplasma fermentans* by means of PCR and found positive for *Mycoplasma fermentans*. On the treatment protocol outlined, all acute CD patients responded by healing and have remained in remission. No post ileo-colectomy cases developed recurrence of CD where this would be expected to occur in 50% of cases.[1] The above results with postoperative clarithromycin reflect an 'open trial' scenario.

In a randomized control trial[10] of antibiotics (metronidazole monotherapy) after ileo-colectomy, considerable reduction of CD occurred but recurrence was not completely eliminated. Clearly antibiotic administration after ileo-colectomy is of benefit.

Non absorbable oral antibiotics such as tobramycin have been used with good effect in ulcerative colitis. A similar ploy has been used for CD. Rifaximin, a semi-synthetic antibiotic used orally to treat traveller's diarrhoea, has been tried in CD. A controlled trial showed remission in moderately active CD[11,12] and similar results were obtained by Shafran in the USA.[13,14]

The overall impression is that antibiotics have great leverage towards improvement of CD. Acute cases of CD and immediate postoperative use of antibiotics appear to give very good therapeutic responses. In a pediatric population antibiotics increase remission of CD with medium term (8 weeks) use of azithromycin and metronidazole.[15]

Questions remain: which bacteria, commensals or pathotypes, and which stage of CD, acute infective or the chronic antigenic phase, are most suitable for the use of antibiotic therapy? Another question is what is the durability of the response to antibiotics in CD.[16] Generally where there is smoke there must be fire. Antibiotics may yet play a role in pinning down a precise cause of CD.

References

1. Selby W, Pavli P, Crotty B et al. Two-year combination therapy with clarithromycin, rifabutin and clofazimine for Crohn's Disease. Gastroenterology 132:2313–2319 (2007)
2. Gui GPH, Thomas PRS, Tizard MIV et al. Two-year-outcomes analysis of Crohn's disease treated with rifabutin and macrolide antibiotics. J Antimicrob Chemo 39:393–400 (1997)
3. Peyrin-Birdulet L, Neut C and Colombel J-F. Antimycobacterial therapy in Crohn's disease: game over? Gastroenterology 132:2594–2598 (2007)
4. Behr MA and Hanley J. Antimycobacterial therapy for Crohn's disease: a reanalysis. Lancet Inf Dis 8:344 (2008)
5. Leiper K, Morris AI and Rhodes JM. Open label trial of oral clarithromycin in active Crohn's disease. Aliment. Pharmacol Ther 14:801–806 (2000)
6. Leiper K, Martin K, Ellis A et al. Clinical trial: randomized study of clarithromycin versus placebo in active Crohn's disease. Aliment Pharmacol Ther 27:1233–1239 (2008)
7. Feller M, Huwiler K, Schoepfer et al. Long term antibiotic treatment for Crohn's disease: systematic review and meta-analysis of placebo-controlled trials. Clin Infect Dis 50:473–80 (2010)
8. Scribano ML and Prantera C. Use of antibiotics in the treatment of Crohn's disease. World J Gastroenterol 19:648–653 (2013)
9. Hannan PCT. Antibiotic susceptibility of *Mycoplasma fermentans* strains from various sources and the development of resistance to aminoglycosides *in vitro*. J Med Microbiol 42:421–428 (1995)
10. Decruz P, Kamm MA, Hamilton AL et al. Crohn's disease management after intestinal resection: a randomized trial. Lancet 385:1406–1417(2015)
11. Prantera C, Lochs H, Campieri M et al. Antibiotic treatment of Crohn's disease results of a multicenter double blind randomized, placebo-controlled trial with rifaximin. Aliment Pharmacol Ther 23:1117–1125 (2006)
12. Prantera C, Lochs H, Grimaldi M et al. Rifaximin-extended intestinal release induced remission in patients with moderately active Crohn's disease. Gastroenterology 142:473–481 (2012)
13. Shafran I and Burgunder P. Rifaximin for the treatment of newly diagnosed Crohn's disease: a case series. Am J Gastroenterol 103:2158–2160 (2008)
14. Shafran I and Burgunder P. Adjunctive antibiotic therapy with rifaximin may help reduce Crohn's Disease activity. Dig Dis Sci 55:1079–1084 (2010)
15. Levine A and Turner D. Combined azithromycin and metronidazole therapy is effective in inducing remission in pediatric Crohn's disease. J Crohns Colitis 5:222–226 (2011)
16. Longman RS and Swaminath A. Microbial manipulation as primary therapy for Crohn's disease. World J Gastroenterol 19:1513–1516 (2013)

PART FOUR

The Road Ahead

-18-

A communality of Colitis

OUTLINE: Nominating the precise type of colitis with the microscope is often difficult and ulcerative-type, Crohn's-type or other-type are often not distinguishable. All forms of colitis display immune cell activation, the activity of which may cloud the precise typing. The communality of colitis is attributed to immune cell activation that follows a communal pathway.

A not unusual problem in the type-diagnosis of colitis by pathologists, looking at tissue samples from the colon, is to assign pathological changes to be either of ulcerative-colitis or Crohn's disease-colitis. An inability to differentiate colitis-types is largely due to a communality of the inflammatory cell response in ulcerative-colitis and Crohn's disease colitis. Of course markers of differentiation in the various forms of colitis exist but these may often not be present. Are there any other forms of colitis in which a 'communality' of immune cell response is shown? Examples are diverticular-colitis and 'colitis by association'.

Diverticular Colitis

This condition arises following an episode of diverticulitis which produces localized colitis either resembling Crohn's disease or ulcerative-colitis. This type of colitis[1] came to the fore with more frequent use of the colonoscope to evaluate the colon after an event of diverticulitis.[2] Following resolution of diverticulitis the colitis is vastly improved, though occasionally an ulcerative colitis-like colitis persists. A key to the cause of diverticular colitis is the active diverticulitis, usually due to a 'blocked' diverticulum from inspissated faecal material. The implication is that the inflammatory cell activation is the key to producing a picture of ulcerative-colitis or Crohn's disease-colitis. The communality of all these colitides are the changes from immune cell activation.

Colitis-by-association

The notion of colitis-by-association derives from clinical observations that attacks of colitis particularly ulcerative-colitis, have an association with upper respiratory tract infections[3] and with seasons.[4] The process involved in colitis-by-association is carriage of nitric oxide by haemoglobin and extraction of nitric oxide into the colon[5] adding to the nitrosative stress that is part of an initial process in the development of colitis (Chapter 7).

Crohn's colitis producing ulcerative colitis

Assuming the proposal that *Mycoplasma fermentans* is causative of Crohn's disease, ulcers in the colonic mucosa would lead to immune cell activation, cytokine production and nitric oxide production by activated macrophages and neutrophils. As mentioned under the causation of ulcerative-colitis (Chapter 7), excessive production of nitric oxide could lead to the development of an ulcerative-colitis-like picture. In this way what started as Crohn's colitis could lead to a picture of ulcerative colitis-like colitis and in fact reflect a combined Crohn's disease-like colitis and ulcerative colitis. Treatment of inflammation may lead to partial resolution of ulcerative colitis-like inflammation but leave the Crohn's disease ulcers. Sequential observations of colitis treatment by the colonoscope would confirm a combined colitis-like picture to have been originally present.

Activated immune cells in Crohn's disease and ulcerative-colitis has been highlighted by Elson in his dissertation on 'immunology of IBD'[6] which has given an admirable picture of the networking of immune cells with consequent production of cytokines, chemokines, eicosanoids and nitric oxide.[7] In immune discussions the 'trigger' for the activation has always remained a question. The answer now given is that in ulcerative-colitis the epithelial barrier is broken down by a concerted and specific production by bacteria of nitric oxide and sulphides, permitting any bacterium to become an immune trigger. In Crohn's disease *Mycoplasma fermentans* in its invasive and antigenic phase due to lipopeptides, is another antigenic trigger. The resultant colitis may be amplified by nitric oxide production from the circulation or an inflamed diverticulum releasing excessive nitric oxide.

The communality of colitis can be attributed to immune cell activation which is very closely patterned despite a variety of antigenic stimuli. Undoubtedly defining the originating trigger to the inflammatory response might lead to better treatment of both Crohn's disease and ulcerative-colitis in the future.

References

1. Evans JP, Cooper J, Roediger WEW. Diverticular colitis – therapeutic and aetiological considerations. Colorectal Dis 4:208–2012(2002)
2. Mulhall AM, Mahid SS, Petras RE et al. Diverticular disease associated with inflammatory bowel disease-like colitis: a systematic review. Dis Colon Rectum 52:1072–1079(2009)
3. Mee AS, Jewell DP. Factors inducing relapse in inflammatory bowel disease. Br Med J 2: 801–802(1978)
4. Moum B, Aadlan DE, Ekbom A et al. Seasonal variation in the onset of ulcerative colitis. Gut 38:376–378(1996)
5. Roediger WEW. Nitric oxide damage to colonocytes in colitis-by-association: remote transfer of nitric oxide to the colon. Digestion 65:191–195(2002)
6. Elson CO. The immunology of inflammatory bowel disease pp. 208–239 in Inflammatory Bowel Disease 5th Ed. Ed JB Kirsner WB Saunders Co, Philadelphia (2000)
7. Knutson CG, Mangerich A, Zeng Y et al. Chemical and cytokine features of innate immunity characterize serum and tissue profiles in inflammatory bowel disease. PNAS 110:E2332-E2341 (2013)

-19-

Future research into the causation of ulcerative colitis and Crohn's disease

OUTLINE: There are many factors in the scope of future research of the causation of ulcerative colitis and Crohn's disease. Measuring in colonic bacteria the genetic profile as well as small molecule production by microbes is needed in ulcerative colitis. Underlying these requisites is a closer study of nitrogen cycling in the colon by dietary means. That *Mycoplasma* are causative of Crohn's disease requires confirmation by prospective studies taking into account the stages of the infective process in Crohn's disease. Scientific dogma and fear-based conformity in science should be relegated so that new views may thrive to more clearly define the causation of ulcerative colitis and Crohn's disease.

Predicting the pathway of future research in inflammatory bowel disease is difficult yet the addition of new thoughts from fresh minds, combined with a determination to proceed to measurement and quantifying observations in patients would provide a means for the task. Scientific creativity needs to be wary that dogmatic ideology, fear-based conformity and institutional inertia are inhibitors of scientific creativity, and these factors need to be overcome.[1]

Ulcerative colitis

We are, in 2016, in an era where the microbiome – the genetic macro assembly of colonic bacteria – has drawn scientists and laboratories to seek answers for disease causation in the human colonic microbiome. Analysis of the genetic profile of the microbiome should in future be in association with assessment of 'small molecule' production by, and stability of, the microbiome[2,3].

In the past, analyses of 'small molecules' of the microbiome have focussed on short chain fatty acids (SCFAs) which have enormous metabolic and physiological leverage in the human colon. A recent re-interpretation of SCFAs is that they regulate immune function of the colonic mucosa and also the ecology of the microbiome.[3] The immunological contentions, newly proposed, are physiologically not very strong at present but views, with further analyses of immune cell capacity, may change in the course of time.

An area of microbial analysis that has lacked traction in humans is the assessment of the capacity of anaerobic respiration in bacteria particularly their role in denitrification. The extent of denitrification may vary extensively in bacteria.[4] Typing bacteria by the capacity of denitrification, the genetic profile and end product analysis (nitrite, nitric oxide and nitrogen gas formation) should bring great dividends in ulcerative colitis. The genes of denitrification in bacteria of soils have been determined (see Chapter 7) but so far not researched in the human microbiome. In short details of nitrogen cycling in the human gut needs a new approach as suggested by Moir[5] and Spiro.[6] Hopefully, pharmaceutical manipulation of the nitrogen cycle by new drugs in ulcerative colitis, will, in future, ameliorate the disease process of ulcerative colitis.

Substrates for bacterial growth in the colon are determined by dietary constituents. The nitrogen content of our diet needs greater attention than in the past. The nitrogen content of food stuffs is variable and is paralleled by the level of protein intake. Further sophisticated dietary studies are needed to help in the treatment of ulcerative colitis.

Crohn's disease

Mycoplasma are frequently detectable in acute Crohn's disease (Chapter 16). Studies to confirm or reject this finding are needed in future. A rapid microbial test for detection of mycoplasma also needs to be developed and attention paid to strain differences in various types of Crohn's disease. Recognition that Crohn's disease is a continuum of a disease process falling into an acute infective phase followed by a chronic antigenic phase requires attention in future-research. At present the terminology in mycoplasmology may not be correct, reflected in past experiences (Chapter 16) and a factor for future exploration. It may emerge that a causative organism for Crohn's disease should be called *Mycoplasma intestinalis*, more accurately reflecting its niche in human anatomy. Such terminology is speculative yet may assign a definite place for mycoplasma in Crohn's disease.

Conclusions

The progress of science is 'tool-driven' through new instrumentation or methodologies and also by new ideas formulated into paradigms.[6] It is important not to relegate 'troublesome' new ideas of disease causation[1] but rather to give support, through development of rhetorical skills of scientists, for future ventures[7]. Peter Doherty in his book *The Knowledge Wars*[8] highlights such a process undertaken successfully with reference to climate change. In general gathering data in inflammatory bowel disease, or climate analysis, is important but the final outcomes depend on the interpretation of the data. The main role of this book was to provide interpretation of data, avoiding dogma, for the observed events in the disease processes of ulcerative colitis and Crohn's disease.

References

1. R. Sheldrake 'The Science Delusion', Hodder and Stoughton, London, (2013)
2. Donia MS and Fischbach MA. Small molecules from the human microbiota. Science 349:395 (2015)
3. Coyte KZ, Schluter J and Foster KR. The ecology of the microbiome: networks, competition and stability. Science 350:663 (2015)
4. Ferguson SJ. Keilins cytochromes: How bacteria use them, vary them and make them. Biochem Soc Trans:29:629–640 (2001)
5. Moir JWB. Bacterial nitrogen cycling in the human body pp. 233–247 in 'Nitrogen Cycling in Bacteria' Molecular Analysis Ed: WB Moir, Caister Academic Press, Norfolk, (2011)
6. Spiro S. Nitric oxide metabolism: physiology and regulatory mechanisms pp. 177–196 in 'Nitrogen Cycling in Bacteria' Molecular Analysis, Caister Academic Press, Norfolk, (2011)
7. Dyson F. The Scientist as Rebel, New York Review Books, New York, (2006)
8. Doherty P. 'The Knowledge Wars' Melbourne University Press, Melbourne (2015)

Appendix

Dietary treatment of ulcerative colitis

Aims of the diet is to diminish the intake of sulphur amino acids from which sulphur for the body is derived. Excess sulphur of the sulphur amino acids that are ingested is transferred back into the colon where sulphides may form. These enhance the damaging effect of nitric oxide.

Avoid completely:	Eggs	
	Cheese	
	Whole milk	
	Ice cream	
	Mayonnaise	
	Cruciferous vegetables:	Cabbage
		Broccoli
		Cauliflower
		Brussel sprouts
	Soya milk	
	Sulphited wines	
	Sulphited cordials	
	Sulphited dried fruit	
Diminish:	Red meat intake	
Use:	Chicken/fish/skimmer milk All other vegetables and complex fibre	

The change in diet takes 4–6 weeks before it becomes effective. Continue with other medication as ordered by your medical advisors.

'Open label' results of the above diet have been published. See Lancet Vol. 351, p. 1555, (1998)

CPSIA information can be obtained
at www.ICGtesting.com
Printed in the USA
BVOW05s0813031017
5983BVAU00004BA/6/P

9 781743 054338